Nurses! Test Yourself in Pathophysiology

T0175984

Nurses! Test Yourself in ...

Titles published in this series:

Nurses! Test Yourself in Anatomy and Physiology, Second Edition
Katherine M. A. Rogers and William N. Scott

Nurses! Test Yourself in Pathophysiology, Second Edition
Katherine M. A. Rogers and William N. Scott

Nurses! Test Yourself in Essential Calculation Skills, Second Edition
Katherine M. A. Rogers and William N. Scott

Nurses! Test Yourself in Pharmacology
Katherine Rogers

Nurses! Test Yourself in Non-medical Prescribing
Noel Harris and Diane Shearer

Nurses! Test Yourself in Clinical Skills
Marian Traynor

Visit www.mcgraw-hill.co.uk/openup/testyourself for further information and sample chapters from other books in the series.

Nurses!
Test Yourself in
Pathophysiology

Second Edition

Katherine M. A. Rogers and William N. Scott

Open University Press

Open University Press
McGraw Hill
Unit 4,
Foundation Park
Roxborough Way
Maidenhead
SL6 3UD

email: emea_uk_ireland@mheducation.com
world wide web: www.mheducation.co.uk

First edition published 2011
First published in this second edition 2024

Executive Editor: Sam Crowe
Editorial Assistant: Hannah Jones
Content Product Manager: Ali Davis

British Library Cataloguing in Publication Data
A catalogue record of this book is available from the British Library

ISBN-13: 9780335250653
ISBN-10: 0335250653
eISBN: 9780335250660

Typeset by Transforma Pvt. Ltd., Chennai, India

Praise page

"I found this updated and refreshed second addition to be a fantastic, contemporary, educational resource. The books structure, combining a systematic, biological systems-based approach, to understanding normal homeostasis, with an in-depth, cellular level consideration of a variety of complex clinical conditions extremely engaging. The book offers the reader valuable insights into understanding patient presentation from a symptoms explanation perspective and addresses, clarifies and demystifies terminology, common clinical investigations and diagnostic tools available to healthcare professionals. The utilisation of a variety of question-and-answer strategies, testing knowledge and understanding, is suitable to a range of learning styles. This new edition offers a fun and flexible learning package that will build confidence when considering the complex pathophysiology field".

Dr Terry J Ferns (EdD) MA BSc (Hons) RN SFHEA, Senior Lecturer, University of Greenwich, UK, Faculty of Education, Health and Human Sciences, London UK

"I have really enjoyed reading this book. I believe it will be a valuable addition for nurses when learning and revising pathophysiology. After an introduction to pathophysiology, abbreviations and relevant terminology the chapters are broken down into systems which help the reader to focus on one system at a time. The chapter content and self-assessment are easily manageable as the design and layout lends itself to learning and revision. Each system is introduced before the reader takes a series of well-constructed multiple-choice questions, puzzles and other self-assessment questions. Answers are then well explained to reinforce learning and allow the reader to correct any areas that they were unsure of. The book then finishes with a useful glossary of terms. I have no hesitation in recommending this book to undergraduate nursing student and will be adding it to the recommended reading list for my undergraduate modules as well as relevant CPD modules."

Conor Hamilton, Lecturer (Education) Nursing, Queen's University Belfast, Ireland

Contents

Acknowledgements

We wish to thank the team at Open University Press for all their help and support throughout the writing of this new edition and those who were involved in the writing of the first edition.

We would also like to acknowledge the reviewers who read our manuscript and provided us with very useful feedback and, of course, the thousands of students we have had the privilege to teach over the years, whose questions and comments have inspired this book (and the other titles in the *Nurses! Test Yourself* series).

We would also like to thank our respective families for their continued patience and support during the writing of this text.

About the authors

Dr Katherine Rogers is a Reader of Bioscience Education at the School of Nursing and Midwifery, Queen's University Belfast. In this role she has been involved in teaching health science subjects – including anatomy, physiology, pathophysiology and pharmacology – from undergraduate to taught doctoral students for over 15 years.

Dr William N. Scott is a Senior Lecturer and Researcher in Biomedicine at Atlantic Technological University. He has been involved in the provision of health and life sciences to undergraduate and postgraduate clinical programmes for many years and has specialist interests in drug discovery and cancer-related fatigue.

Katherine and William are also external examiners in these subjects for several Higher Education Institutions across the UK, Ireland and internationally, and have authored and edited numerous textbooks and peer-reviewed articles. Together, they are Editors of the *Nurses! Test Yourself* series.

Using this book

INTRODUCTION

Welcome to the second edition of *Nurses! Test Yourself in Pathophysiology*. We hope you continue to find this an invaluable tool throughout your pathophysiology course and beyond!

This book is designed to be used as a revision aid that you can use with your main learning resources (such as lecture notes and textbook). Each chapter is designed for stand-alone revision, meaning that you need not read from the beginning to benefit from the book – you can dip in and out as you need to.

Every chapter begins with a brief introduction covering the main points of the topic and directing you to some useful resources. The chapter progresses, providing you with different types of questions that help you test your knowledge of the area. These are:

- *Labelling exercise*: identify the different elements on the diagram.
- *True or false*: identify if the statement is true or false.
- *Multiple choice*: identify which of four answers is correct.
- *Fill in the blanks*: fill in the blanks to complete the statement.
- *Match the terms*: identify which term matches which statement.
- *Puzzle grids*: use the word banks and clues to solve the word puzzle.

The questions have been designed to be slightly more challenging in each section. Do not ignore a question type just because you are not tested in that way because the answer contains useful information that could easily be examined in an alternative question format.

Answers are provided in each chapter with detailed explanations – this is to help you with revision but can also be used as a learning aid. In certain answers you will find hints, tips, mnemonics or acronyms, to aid revision and recall. We find that students particularly like these pointers as they help with learning, so feel free to come up with your own as well!

A list of common abbreviations used throughout the book and a list of common prefixes, suffixes and word roots commonly used in pathophysiology are provided. At the back there is a glossary.

We have suggested some useful textbooks that may be used to support your recommended text, but they should not replace the core reading for your course.

We hope that you enjoy using this book and that you find it a convenient and useful tool throughout your studies!

GUIDE TO TEXTBOOK RESOURCES

Nurses! Test Yourself in Anatomy and Physiology, 2nd edition,
Katherine M. A. Rogers and William N. Scott
Published by McGraw-Hill, 2021

Fluids and Electrolytes Made incredibly Easy, 1st edition,
William N. Scott
Published by Lippincott, Williams & Wilkins, 2010

Fundementals of Applied Pathophysiology: An Essential Guide for Nursing and Healthcare Students, 4th edition,
Ian Peate
Published by Wiley-Blackwell, 2021

Gould's Pathophysiology for the Healthcare Professions, 7th edition,
Karin C. VanMeter and Robert J Hubert
Published by Elsevier, 2022

Ross and Wilson's Anatomy and Physiology in Health and Illness, 14th edition,
Anne Waugh and Alison Grant
Published by Churchill Livingstone, 2022

Symptoms, Diagnosis and Treatment, 1st edition,
Paul Rutter
Published by Churchill Livingstone, 2005

List of abbreviations

These are common abbreviations used in the clinical setting and throughout this book.

ABG	arterial blood gas	**CT**	computerized tomography
ACE	angiotensin-converting enzyme	**CTS**	carpal tunnel syndrome
		CVA	cerebrovascular accident (or stroke)
ACS	acute coronary syndrome		
ADH	antidiuretic hormone (or vasopressin)	**CVD**	cardiovascular disease
		CVS	chorionic villus sampling
AIDS	acquired immunodeficiency syndrome	**DEXA**	dual energy X-ray absorptiometry
ALL	acute lymphocytic leukaemia	**DI**	diabetes insipidus
		DKA	diabetic ketoacidosis
AML	acute myeloid leukaemia	**DM**	diabetes mellitus
ASD	autistic spectrum disorders	**DRE**	digital rectal examination
AST	aspartate aminotransferase	**DVT**	deep vein thrombosis
BP	blood pressure	**ECG**	electrocardiogram
BUN	blood urea nitrogen	**EEG**	electroencephalogram
CAD	coronary artery disease	**EMG**	electromyography
CF	cystic fibrosis	**ERCP**	endoscopic retrograde cholangio-pancreatography
CK	creatinine kinase		
CKD	chronic kidney disease (end-stage renal disease)		
		ESWL	extracorporeal shock wave lithotripsy
CLL	chronic lymphocytic leukaemia	**FH**	familial hypercholesterolaemia
CML	chronic myeloid leukaemia		
CO$_2$	carbon dioxide	**GCS**	Glasgow Coma Scale
COPD	chronic obstructive pulmonary disorders (or diseases)	**GFR**	glomerular filtration rate
		GI	gastrointestinal
		GP	general practitioner
CRF	chronic renal failure	**GTN**	glyceryl trinitrate
CSF	cerebrospinal fluid	**HDL**	high-density lipoprotein

HDU	high dependency unit	**O₂**	oxygen
HIV	human immunodeficiency virus	**PCNL**	percutaneous nephrolithotomy
HNPCC	hereditary non-polyposis colorectal cancer	**PD**	Parkinson's disease
HPV	human papilloma virus	**PEFR**	peak expiratory flow rate
HRT	hormone replacement therapy	**PID**	pelvic inflammatory disease
HSV	herpes simplex virus	**PKU**	phenylketonuria
ICP	intracranial pressure	**PPI**	proton-pump inhibitor
ICU	intensive care unit	**PSA**	prostate-specific antigen
IDDM	insulin-dependent diabetes mellitus	**RBC**	red blood cell (or erythrocyte)
IV	intravenous	**RIRS**	retrograde intrarenal surgery
IVP	intravenous pyelogram	**SAH**	subarachnoid haemorrhage
IVU	intravenous urogram		
LAD	lactate dehydrogenase	**SCLC**	small-cell lung cancer
LDL	low-density lipoprotein	**SOB**	shortness of breath
LP	lumbar puncture (or spinal tap)	**STEMI**	ST-elevation myocardial infarction
MI	myocardial infarction (or heart attack)	**STI**	sexually transmitted infection
mM	millimolar	**TIA**	transient ischaemic attack (or 'mini-stroke')
mmol/L	millimoles per litre		
MRI	magnetic resonance imaging	**TSH**	thyroid-stimulating hormone
Non-STEMI	non-ST-elevation myocardial infarction	**UTI**	urinary tract infection
		UV	ultra-violet
NSAID	non-steroidal anti-inflammatory drug	**VTE**	venous thromboembolism
NSCLC	non-small-cell lung cancer	**WBC**	white blood cell (or leukocyte)

Directional terms

Abduct	move away from the midline of the body; the opposite of adduct
Adduct	movement towards the midline of the body; the opposite of abduct
Anterior	front-facing or ventral; opposite of posterior or dorsal
Contralateral	on opposite side; opposite of ipsilateral
Distal	far away from point of origin; the opposite of proximal
Dorsal	to the back or posterior of; opposite of ventral or anterior
Inferior	lower or beneath; opposite to superior
Ipsilateral	on same side; opposite to contralateral
Lateral	referring to the side, away from the midline; opposite of medial
Medial	towards the middle; opposite of lateral
Posterior	back or dorsal; opposite of anterior or ventral
Proximal	nearest to the centre of the body; opposite of distal
Superior	above or higher; opposite of inferior
Ventral	referring to front or anterior; opposite of dorsal or posterior

The table below summarizes how these terms match up.

Direction	Opposite term
Abduct	Adduct
Anterior/ventral	Posterior/dorsal
Contralateral	Ipsilateral
Distal	Proximal
Inferior	Superior
Lateral	Medial

Common prefixes, suffixes and roots

Prefix/suffix/root	Definition	Example
a-/an-	deficiency, lack of	anuria = decrease or absence of urine production
-aemia	of the blood	ischaemia = decreased blood supply
angio-	vessel	angiogenesis = growth of new vessels
broncho-	bronchus	bronchitis = inflammation of the bronchus
card-	heart	cardiology = study of the heart
chole-	bile or gall bladder	cholecystitis = inflammation of gall bladder
cyto-	cell	cytology = study of cells
derm-	skin	dermatology = study of the skin
entero-	intestine	enteritis = inflammation of the intestinal tract
erythro-	red	erthyropenia = deficiency of red blood cells
gast-	stomach	gastritis = inflammation of stomach lining
-globin	protein	haemoglobin = iron-containing protein in the blood
haem-	blood	haemocyte = a blood cell (especially red blood cell)
hepat-	liver	hepatitis = inflammation of the liver
-hydr-	water	rehydrate = replenish body fluids
leuko-	white	leukopenia = deficiency of white blood cells
lymph-	lymph tissue/vessels	lymphoedema = fluid retention in lymphatic system
myo-	muscle	myocardium = cardiac muscle
nephr-	kidney	nephritis = inflammation of the kidneys
neuro-	nerve	neurology = study of the nerves
-ology	study of	histology = study of the tissues
-ophth-	eye	ophthalmology = study of the eyes
osteo-	bone	osteology = study of bones
path-	disease	pathology = study of disease
pneumo-	air/lungs	pneumonitis = inflammation of lung tissue
-uria	urine	haematuria = blood in the urine
vaso-	vessel	vasoconstriction = narrowing of vessels

1 Introduction to pathophysiology

INTRODUCTION

The body is always striving to maintain an internal equilibrium called homeostasis, which is regulated by the brain and maintained by a number of positive and negative feedback mechanisms. Disease or illness may develop when homeostasis is disrupted. The study of pathophysiology (or pathobiology) relates to the changes that occur in normal anatomy and physiology as a result of illness or disease.

A key principle of anatomy and physiology is that cells are the building blocks of the body; the body is made up of organs, which consist of a collection of tissues, and these are made up of cells. Therefore, any cellular change or damage can affect the whole body. An analogy to consider is the foundations of a building: if the foundations are unstable or damaged, then the whole building is at risk of collapse; similarly, if cells (or their contents) are damaged or not functioning properly, then the structure and/or function of the tissues, organs and whole body may also be affected because the cells are the building blocks of the whole body.

Injury, malnutrition or invasion by pathogens can all disrupt homeostasis. Cells check for such imbalances during replication and usually adapt successfully in response to such stresses. However, sometimes the dividing cell fails to detect unwanted changes and the resulting mutation(s) may cause disease.

In the study of pathophysiology, we usually consider a number of factors: the causes of disease (aetiology), the changes to normal anatomy and physiology (pathophysiology), the signs and symptoms (clinical manifestations) of the disease or illness, along with diagnostic tests and treatments available.

This chapter examines changes in homeostasis and how this leads to illness or disease. To assess a patient's symptoms and be able to plan, deliver and evaluate their care, nurses need to understand how changes to normal anatomy and physiology at a cell and tissue level are associated with both the local and systemic signs and symptoms of various disease processes.

Useful resources

Nurses! Test Yourself in Anatomy and Physiology (2nd edition)
Chapter 1

Ross and Wilson's Anatomy and Physiology in Health and Illness (14th edition)
Chapters 1 and 3

LABELLING EXERCISE

1–7 The structure of normal cells is shown as a guide in Figure 1.1. Each of the other diagrams represents a type of cellular change. Compare each diagram of cellular change against the normal cells shown and identify the cellular adaptations using the terms in the box below.

hyperplasia	severe dysplasia	atrophy
mild dysplasia	metastasis	hypertrophy
metaplasia		

Figure 1.1 Cellular adaptations

Normal cells

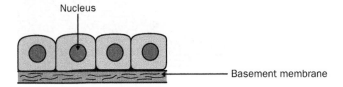

1. _____

2. _____

3. _____

4. _____

5. _____

6. _____

7. _____

TRUE OR FALSE?

Are the following statements true or false?

8   There are four types of homeostatic feedback mechanisms.

9   Disease can develop when normal homeostasis cannot be sustained.

10   The division of somatic cells involves three stages.

11   A biopsy is a medical procedure that involves a healthcare practitioner removing a small sample of body tissue for examination under a microscope.

12   Cancer is a condition that develops when cells die uncontrollably.

13   During their lifetime, cells face constant challenges to their normal function.

14   When assessing pain, remember the acronym PQRST.

MULTIPLE CHOICE

Identify one correct answer for each of the following:

15 Homeostasis can be defined as:

a) functional changes caused by disease

b) an unbalanced state, out of equilibrium

c) a steady, dynamic state of equilibrium

d) the exaggeration of an original response

16 How many components are there in a homeostatic feedback mechanism?

a) 6

b) 5

c) 4

d) 3

17 Which of the following regions of the brain is *not* involved in maintaining homeostasis?

a) pons

b) medulla oblongata

c) pituitary gland

d) reticular formation

18 What is the name of the process that describes the transformation from a normal cell to a cancerous cell?

a) carcinogenesis

b) replication

c) mutation

d) necrosis

19 Most solid cancerous tumours arise from which type of tissue?

a) glandular

b) skin

c) nervous

d) epithelial

FILL IN THE BLANKS

Fill in the blanks in each statement using the options in this box.
Not all of them are required, so choose carefully!

chronic	tissue	pathology
metastasize	residual	acute
latent	pathogenesis	contagious
organ	remission	referred
carcinogenesis	illness	aetiology

20 The _____ of a disease can be intrinsic or extrinsic.

21 The development of a disease is called its _____.

22 Complete the stages in disease progression:

    i)   injury/exposure

    ii) _____ phase

    iii) prodromal period

    iv) _____ phase

    v) _____

    vi) convalescence

    vii) recovery

23 Cytology and histology are branches of _____ .

24 The pain radiating along the left arm often reported by MI patients is called _____ pain.

25 A solid tumour is usually classified according to the _____ from which it originates.

26 Cancer cells can _____ away from their origin.

PUZZLE GRID

Use the word bank (below) and clues (overleaf) to solve the puzzle.

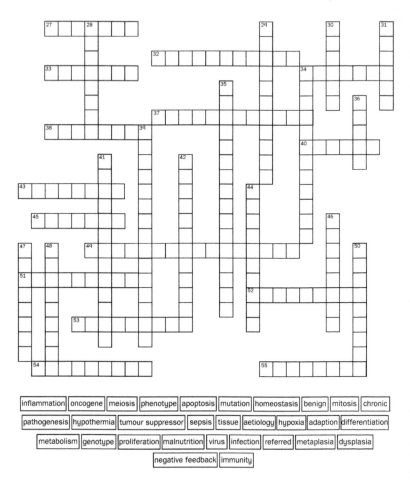

inflammation	oncogene	meiosis	phenotype	apoptosis	mutation	homeostasis	benign	mitosis	chronic
pathogenesis	hypothermia	tumour suppressor	sepsis	tissue	aetiology	hypoxia	adaption	differentiation
metabolism	genotype	proliferation	malnutrition	virus	infection	referred	metaplasia	dysplasia
negative feedback	immunity

Clues across

27   Deprivation of an adequate oxygen supply at the tissue level (7)

32   Abnormally low core body temperature (11)

33   Process of cell division occurring in somatic cells (7)

34   Division of germ cells resulting in haploid cell formation (7)

37   Generic response to tissue injury characterized by heat, redness, pain, swelling and loss of function (12)

38   Type of pain located away from, or adjacent to, the organ involved (8)

40   Group of structurally and functionally similar cells (6)

43   Permanent change in the genome resulting from alterations in DNA nucleotide sequences (8)

45   Description of long-lasting conditions such as diabetes, osteoporosis or cardiac disease (7)

49   Important type of control mechanism associated with homeostasis (8, 8)

51   Transformation of one differentiated cell type to another (10)

52   Invasion of body tissues by parasitic organisms or opportunistic pathogens (9)

53   Programmed cell death occurring throughout tissue during normal development and ageing (9)

54   Presence of abnormal cells within a tissue or organ that may progress to cancer (9)

55   The genetic makeup of a cell that contributes to its phenotype (8)

Clues down

28   Mutated form of a gene involved in cell proliferation that may cause the growth of neoplasms (8)

29   Self-regulating process by which the body maintains a relatively constant internal environment (11)

30   Used to describe a disease or condition having little or no detrimental effect (6)

31   Life-threatening organ dysfunction caused by a dysregulated host response to infection (6)

34   Imbalance resulting from deficiency or excess of dietary components (12)

35   Class of gene involved in the inhibition of cellular proliferation; anti-oncogene (6, 10)

36   Obligate intracellular parasite (5)

39   Process by which cells, tissue and organs acquire specialized features (15)

41   Rapid growth or reproduction of cells (13)

42   Mechanism and process by which a disease develops (12)

44   Set of cellular reactions that are set to maintain life; includes both anabolism and catabolism (10)

46   Mechanism by which cells and tissues adjust to an altered environment (8)

47   Term that describes sufficient biological defences to avoid infection or disease (8)

48   Causative factors of a condition or disease (9)

50   Physical appearance or characteristics of the genotype; observable traits (9)

ANSWERS

LABELLING EXERCISE

Figure 1.2 Cellular Adaptations

Normal cells

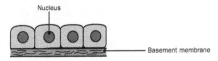

Nucleus

Basement membrane

1.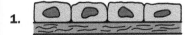

2.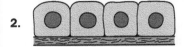

3.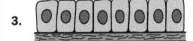

4.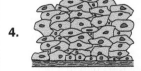

5.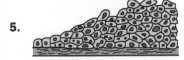

6.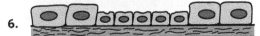

7.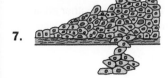

Normal human cells come in many shapes and sizes; their shapes change as they differentiate and adopt specialized functions – for example, a red blood cell looks very different to a muscle or nerve cell. When examined through a microscope, different cell types do not look alike; however, cells of the same type will appear very similar, with a uniform size and shape, and a regular pattern of arrangement.

1 *Atrophy* refers to the reversible reduction or shrinkage in cell size. It can happen when cells are no longer used, are malnourished, have insufficient blood supply, lack of innervation or have insufficient hormonal stimulation. The shrinkage in size of the thymus gland in adults is an example of normal atrophy due to disuse. Note that the atrophied cells are smaller than the normal cells (shown in Figure 1.2 for comparison).

2 *Hypertrophy* describes an increase in cell size rather than increase in the number of cells. (*Hint*: the suffix *-trophy* usually refers to size). Note that these cells are larger than the normal cells.

3 *Hyperplasia* is an increase in the number of cells caused by increased workload, hormonal stimulation or decreased tissue. It differs from metaplasia, which describes replacement of cells rather than an increase in cell number. (*Hint*: the suffix *-plasia* usually refers to formation or growth). Note there are many more cells occupying the same space compared to the normal cells.

4 *Mild dysplasia* describes abnormal growth or development of tissues or cells, leading to a change in size, shape and appearance that is sometimes reversible but often precedes neoplastic (cancerous) changes. Note how these cells have lost the uniform shape and arrangement of the normal cells.

5 *Severe dysplasia (carcinoma in situ)* describes a group of abnormal cells that are found only in the place where they first formed (primary location) and have not spread to other parts of the body. Carcinoma *in situ* is often considered to be the earliest form of cancer development.

6 *Metaplasia* is the replacement of one adult cell with another adult cell that can better endure some change or stress. It is usually a response to chronic inflammation or irritation.

7 | ***Metastasis (invasive carcinoma)*** In metastasis, cancer cells break away from the site where they first formed (known as the primary tumour) and spread to other areas of the body, usually via the blood or lymphatic system, forming a new tumour (called a metastatic tumour) in other organs or tissues in other parts of the body. The new, metastatic tumour is the same type of cancer as the primary tumour. For example, if breast cancer spreads to the lung, the cancer cells in the lung are usually identifiable as breast cancer cells, not lung cancer cells. This is useful when diagnosing cancers and determining if a tumour is a primary or secondary neoplasm. (See Answer 26).

TRUE OR FALSE?

8 | **There are four types of homeostatic feedback mechanisms.**
The *two* types of feedback mechanisms are: positive feedback and negative feedback. Positive feedback occurs when a stimulus triggers an enhanced response exaggerating the original event. Negative feedback mechanisms restore homeostasis by detecting and correcting changes to the normal homeostatic conditions in the body. There are fewer examples of positive feedback than negative feedback; examples include platelet formation in the blood coagulation cascade (haemostasis) and oxytocin release during labour contractions in childbirth. Examples of negative feedback include secretion of insulin from the pancreas to reduce high blood sugar levels back to normal, control of body temperature by thermoreceptors in the hypothalamus (thermoregulation), and control of blood pressure and respiration rate.

9 | **Disease can develop when normal homeostasis cannot be sustained.**
A disease will usually induce specific signs and symptoms that may require investigation. Disease develops following disruption of the body's normal homeostasis, while illness describes poor health caused by disease. Disease differs from illness because an individual may live a reasonably normal life and not be considered ill, despite having a disease. For example, an asthmatic person can live a normal life and not usually be considered ill because the body

has adapted to the disease. However, the disease may make them more susceptible to certain illnesses such as respiratory infections or pneumonia.

10   **The division of somatic cells involves three stages.**
Somatic cell division has *two* stages. The first stage is mitosis, when the nucleus and genetic material of the cell divide. In mitosis, there are a number of different growth and synthesis phases. The second stage in cell reproduction is cytokinesis. At the beginning of this stage the cytoplasm divides; it ends when the new cell's contents divides into two new daughter cells (by convention, new cells are called daughter cells). In gametes (sex cells), cell division and reproduction occur by meiosis.

11   **A biopsy is a medical procedure that involves a healthcare practitioner removing a small sample of body tissue for examination under a microscope.**
A tissue sample may be excised from almost anywhere inside or on the surface the body, including the skin, organs and other structures. There are several different types of biopsies and the type used will depend on the area of the body that requires the investigation. A biopsy is often associated with cancer diagnostics; however, a biopsy can be used to identify many other conditions. Biopsies usually involve removing larger pieces of tissue than a cytology, and a pathologist may examine several types of cells in a tissue sample taken from a biopsy. Biopsy procedures are also generally more invasive than cytology tests and may require local or general anaesthesia to reduce pain or discomfort for the patient.

12   **Cancer is a condition that develops when cells die uncontrollably.** **X**
Cancer develops due to excessive and uncontrollable cell growth. A cancerous (or neoplastic) cell develops due to a mutation of a single gene which affects the control of normal function in the cell. The mutation allows the cell to grow and proliferate without the normal regulatory controls of cell growth and replication and it loses the ability to enter apoptosis (programmed cell death). Initially, the uncontrolled growth of the cancerous cells is localized but because they have lost the ability to perform apoptosis, the cells do not die and so the mass of proliferating cells begins to invade nearby tissue and may eventually metastasize

to other areas of the body. Most cancers are solid tumours but malignancies can arise in the blood – these are called haematological cancers. Necrosis is an undesirable form of cell death usually caused by factors external to the cell, such as trauma, toxins or infection.

13 **During their lifetime, cells face constant challenges to their normal function.**
The normal functioning of the cell is constantly being challenged by stressors within the body and its external environment. The cell can normally adapt to such stressors and continue to function normally. However, sometimes the cell is unable to adapt to these challenges allowing stressors to induce changes to the body's state of health, causing disease or illness. When cells are stressed, they can undergo a number of changes: atrophy, hypertrophy, hyperplasia, metaplasia or dysplasia (see Figure 1.2).

14 **When assessing pain, remember the acronym PQRST.**
PQRST is a useful prompt to remember what questions to ask a patient when assessing pain.

P = *precipitation/palliation*– what causes the pain and what relieves it?
Q = *quality* – how could the pain be described, is it crushing, dull, sharp or stabbing?
R = *region/radiation* – where did the pain start and has it spread elsewhere?
S = *severity* – how bad is the pain, using a scale of 0 = no pain to 10 = worst pain?
T = *timing*– when did the pain start and how long does it last?

MULTIPLE CHOICE
Correct answers identified in *bold italics*

15 **Homeostasis can be defined as:**
a) functional changes caused by disease
b) an unbalanced state, out of equilibrium
c) *a steady, dynamic state of equilibrium*
d) the exaggeration of an original response

Homeostasis involves intricate and tightly controlled events that the body uses to preserve the stability of the internal environment of cells, tissues, organs and systems and hence helps keep the body in good health. Homeostasis helps to maintain the volume and temperature of body fluids so that the body exists in a favourable environment to remain healthy. It is controlled by the brain and is regulated by positive and negative feedback mechanisms. The hallmark of the ageing process is a decrease in the body's ability to maintain homeostasis because the body becomes less able to adapt to stressors. For example, many individuals suffer from hypertension as they get older because the blood vessels lose elasticity and therefore are less able to adapt to changes in blood pressure.

16 **How many components are there in a homeostatic feedback mechanism?**

a) 6   b) 5   c) 4   *d)* **3**

Every homeostatic feedback mechanism has three components: (1) a sensory mechanism – to detect deviations in the homeostatic equilibrium; (2) a control centre in the central nervous system – which regulates the body's response to the change; and (3) an effector mechanism – which receives responses from the CNS that help restore homeostatic equilibrium.

17 **Which of the following regions of the brain is *not* involved in maintaining homeostasis?**

a) *pons*   b)   medulla oblongata
c)   pituitary gland   d)   reticular formation

Three parts of the brain are involved in maintaining homeostasis in the body. They are the medulla oblongata (in the brain stem), the pituitary gland (at the base of the brain, directly above the hypothalamus) and the reticular formation (located deep within the brain stem). The medulla oblongata controls a number of vital functions such as circulation and respiration. The pituitary gland controls the function of other glands and is involved in regulation of growth, maturation and reproduction. The reticular formation is a group of nerve cells that control certain vital reflexes such as cardiovascular function and respiration. The pons is located just above the medulla oblongata but is not involved in maintaining homeostasis.

It houses several cranial nerves that are involved in interpreting sensory information.

18 **What is the name of the process that describes the transformation from a normal cell to a cancerous cell?**

a) *carcinogenesis*　　　b) replication
c) mutation　　　　　　　d) necrosis

There is no single cause that triggers carcinogenesis. It is likely to be induced by a number of triggers that interact together and that the cell is unable to defend against. These triggers can be genetic, lifestyle factors (smoking, diet, lack of exercise), hormonal, metabolic, viral, radiation or chemical in nature. Carcinogenesis is a multi-stage process that involves a pre-clinical (latent) phase and a clinical phase. In some cancers, the latent phase can last for many years and in others it may be very short (weeks, months). The main stages of carcinogenesis include:

I. *initiation* – the introduction of a spontaneous or induced genetic mutation;

II. *promotion* – confers a selective growth advantage that allows the abnormal cell to grow and proliferate;

III. *progression* – a series of additional mutations allow the mutated cell to continue to grow and evade apoptosis - cells may not be distinguishable from the parent cell;

IV. *metastatic spread* – the movement of cancerous cells away from their site of origin.

19 **The majority of solid cancerous tumours arise from:**

a) glandular tissue　　　b) skin tissue
c) nervous tissue　　　　*d)* *epithelial tissue*

Any cancer derived from epithelial tissue is usually classified as a carcinoma. Cancers derived from glandular tissue are called adenocarcinomas. Tumours of the nervous tissue are termed gliomas. Tumours derived from supporting tissue such as muscle, bone and connective tissues are called sarcomas. Lymphatic and immune system tumours are classified as lymphomas. Tumours of the white blood cells are leukaemias, while tumours of the pigment cells are called melanomas. Plasma cell tumours are classified as myelomas.

FILL IN THE BLANKS

20 **The *aetiology* of a disease can be intrinsic or extrinsic.**
The aetiology (or cause) of a disease can be influenced by the individual's biochemistry (intrinsic) or environmental (extrinsic) factors. Intrinsic biochemical factors are beyond an individual's control since they include such things as age, gender and genetics. Extrinsic factors are influenced by lifestyle and the external environment. They can include stress, diet, drug use (prescribed and illicit), smoking, injury, bacteria or viral infections, exposure to chemical or radioactive agents, and exposure to extreme temperatures. Occasionally, diseases arise that have no known aetiology - these are described as idiopathic.

21 **The development of a disease is called its *pathogenesis*.**
Most diseases have defined symptoms of progression that they will follow if left untreated. Some diseases are described as *self-limiting* because they resolve themselves without any interventions; other diseases will never resolve and are described as chronic. Patients with chronic diseases may experience periods of remission or exacerbation. During remission, symptoms improve or disappear while during exacerbation a patient may suffer increasing severity of symptoms. An example of a chronic condition that can undergo such periods is the inflammatory disease, rheumatoid arthritis.

22 **Complete the stages in disease progression:**
i)   injury/exposure
ii) *latent* phase
iii) prodromal period
iv) *acute* phase
v)   *remission*
vi) convalescence
vii) recovery

A disease progresses through a number of stages in the order described (i to vii) and is triggered by an injury or exposure to a pathogen. During the latent or incubation period, no signs or symptoms will be observed. During the prodromal period, mild signs and symptoms will be observed but are usually non-specific (such as headache, nausea, fever). In the acute phase, the disease is at its peak; complications may arise in this phase. If the patient is still able to function in a reasonably normal manner, this phase may be called a subclinical acute phase. Remission is a second latent phase and occurs after the disease has reached its peak. It may be followed by a relapse into another acute phase. During convalescence, the disease has passed and the patient progresses towards recovery. A patient is said to be recovered when there are no signs and symptoms of disease. At this stage, the patient has generally returned to normal health.

23 **Cytology and histology are branches of _pathology_.**
Pathology is a branch of medicine that involves laboratory examination of cells in samples of body tissue or fluids for diagnostic purposes. Cytology usually involves examining individual cells or clusters of cells through a microscope. Pathologists usually need a very small sample of cells for cytology tests, thus these types of tests are usually relatively painless, although some patients may experience mild discomfort during the procedure. A common example of a cytology screening test is a cervical smear test. Histology is the examination of an entire section of tissue, which contains many types of cells. Depending on the tissue type, disease processes can affect tissues in distinctive ways. Histopathology (the study of tissues affected by disease) tests are very useful for making a diagnosis and may also be helpful when determining the severity and progression of disease.

24 **The pain radiating along the left arm often reported by MI patients is called _referred_ pain.**
Referred (or reflective) pain describes pain experienced in part of the body at a distance from its area of origin. The mechanisms of referred pain are not fully understood, but is thought to happen when nerve fibres from various regions or organs converge on the same levels of the spinal cord. The best-known example is pain experienced during a myocardial infarction. Nerves from damaged cardiac tissue convey pain signals to spinal cord levels T1–T4 on the left side, which are the same levels that receive sensation from the left side of the chest and part of the left arm. This very close proximity of the converging nerve fibres confuses the brain, which interprets the heart pain as coming from the chest area and left

arm (and sometimes the neck or jaw). Figure 1.3 illustrates common areas where referred pain may be experienced.

Figure 1.3 Referred pain regions

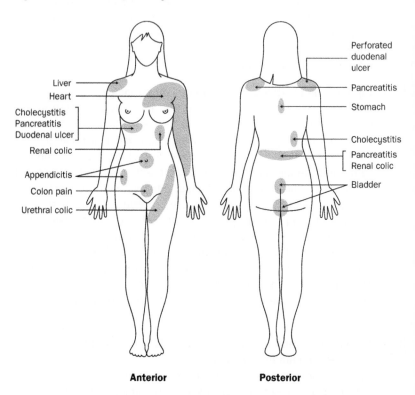

Liver
Heart
Cholecystitis
Pancreatitis
Duodenal ulcer
Renal colic
Appendicitis
Colon pain
Urethral colic

Perforated duodenal ulcer
Pancreatitis
Stomach
Cholecystitis
Pancreatitis
Renal colic
Bladder

Anterior   **Posterior**

25 | **A solid tumour is usually classified according to the _tissue_ from which it originates.**
The majority of solid tumours arise from epithelial tissue, which is the main type of tissue that lines the internal and external surfaces of the body's organs (for example, the lungs, colon and breasts). Tumours arising from epithelial tissues are called carcinomas. Haematological cancers are classified according to the blood cells from which they originate.

26 **Cancer cells can _metastasize_ away from their origin.**

The metastasis of cancer cells is the movement or spread of the cells to other areas of the body (see Answer 7) and may occur in three ways:

I. The growing mass of cells penetrates a blood or lymphatic vessel, enters the circulating blood or lymph and travels through either system. The cells can then settle in any organ or region of the body and establish secondary tumours with pathological characteristics similar to the primary cancer tumour. Some types of cancer have locations to which they commonly metastasize.

II. Cancerous cells can be spread during surgery.

III. They can spread to neighbouring organs – this is common in the GI tract because of the close proximity of organs.

There are many pathophysiological changes associated with the development of metastases. Sometimes it is only through the detection of such metastatic signs and symptoms that a cancer is diagnosed. Some common clinical signs of metastases include pleural effusion of the lungs, which may indicate a metastasis in the lungs – a common metastatic site for breast cancers (or it may be indicative of a primary lung tumour); ascites in the peritoneum can indicate metastasis in the peritoneal cavity, which is a common metastatic site for ovarian cancers.

PUZZLE GRID

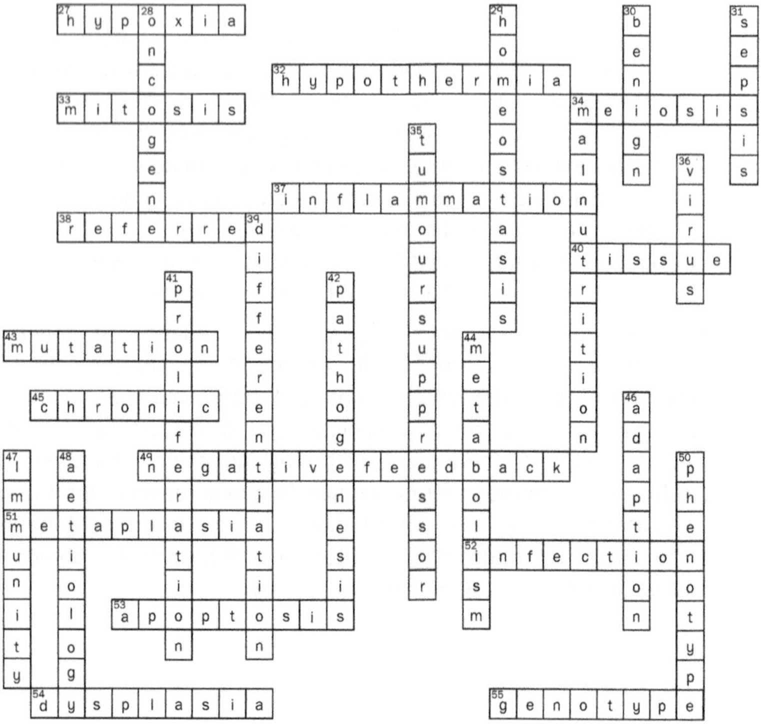
27 hypoxia
28 oncogen
29 homeostasis
30 benign
31 sepsis
32 hypothermia
33 mitosis
34 meiosis
34 malnutrition
35 tumoursuppressor
36 virus
37 inflammation
38 referred
39 differentiation
40 tissue
41 proliferation
42 pathogenesis
43 mutation
44 metabolism
45 chronic
46 adaptation
47 immunity
48 aetiology
49 negativefeedback
50 phenotype
51 metaplasia
52 infection
53 apoptosis
54 dysplasia
55 genotype

2 Inflammation, infection and immunity

INTRODUCTION

The immune system has three lines of defence: (1) physical and chemical barriers against infective agents; (2) the inflammatory response; and (3) the immune system reaction. When pathogens invade the body, there are two types of possible immune response that can occur: specific and non-specific.

Infection occurs when the body's defence mechanisms are invaded by pathogens. Inflammation is a protective attempt by the body to remove the inflammatory stimulus and initiate the healing process in the tissue. Inflammation can be classified as either acute or chronic. Acute inflammation is the body's initial response to harmful stimuli, while chronic (prolonged) inflammation causes a change in the type of cells present at the inflammation site. In the absence of inflammation, wounds and infections would never heal, causing progressive destruction of the tissue.

Immunodeficiency occurs when the immune system is less functional than normal, resulting in recurring and life-threatening infections. In contrast, autoimmune diseases are caused by a hyperactive immune system that attacks normal tissues as if they were foreign organisms. Hypersensitivity disorders are often caused by an overactive immune response.

Nurses need to recognize the characteristics of infection and inflammation to treat such conditions quickly and efficiently because certain infections can develop rapidly and be life-threatening.

Useful resources

Nurses! Test Yourself in Anatomy and Physiology (2nd edition)
Chapter 12

Ross and Wilson's Anatomy and Physiology in Health and Illness (14th edition)
Chapter 15

TRUE OR FALSE?

Are the following statements true or false?

| 1 | Disorders of the immune system fall into three main categories. |

| 2 | Inflammation is classified in three main ways. |

| 3 | An organism that causes an infection in the human body by evading the immune system is called a pathogen. |

| 4 | For infection control, nurses should always wear gloves during patient contact. |

| 5 | Bacteria contain carbohydrates that may cause infection. |

| 6 | Fungi can be classified as yeasts or moulds. |

| 7 | Parasitic infections are very common in cold climates. |

| 8 | B-cells are responsible for humoral immunity. |

MULTIPLE CHOICE

Identify one correct answer for each of the following:

9 Which of the following is *not* a sign of inflammation?

a) heat

b) improvement/gain of function

c) pain

d) redness

10 Tonsillitis is most commonly caused by:

a) viruses

b) bacteria

c) fungi

d) protozoa

11 Pathogens can be transmitted via which of the following routes?

a) airborne

b) arthropods

c) direct and indirect contact

d) all of the above

12 Which of the following is a major protein cascade that supports the inflammatory response?

a) inflammation system

b) complimentary system

c) complement system

d) compliment system

FILL IN THE BLANKS

Fill in the blanks in each statement using the options in this box.
Not all of them are required, so choose carefully!

opportunistic	viral	T-
infection	carcinogenesis	B-
latent		

13 _____ can occur when a pathogen or disease-causing substance enters the body.

14 _____ infections occur when normal immune and inflammatory responses fail.

15 _____ infections usually occur in people with weakened immune systems.

16 In the cell-mediated immune response, _____ cells respond directly to the foreign antigen.

MATCH THE TERMS

Classify each immune disorder listed below:

A. autoimmune   **B. hypersensitivity**

C. immunodeficiency

---

17 Anaphylaxis _____

18 HIV disease _____

19 Rheumatoid arthritis _____

20 Lupus erythematosus _____

21 Allergic rhinitis _____

PUZZLE GRID

Use the word bank (below) and clues (overleaf) to solve the puzzle.

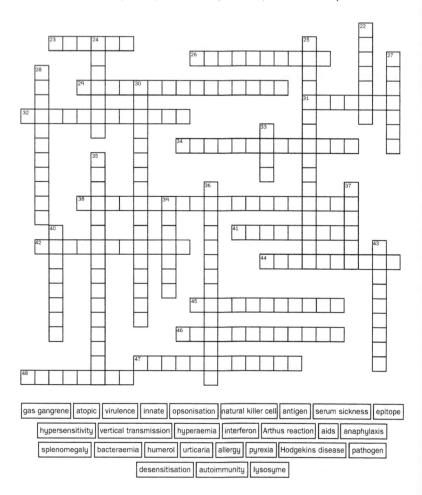

| gas gangrene | atopic | virulence | innate | opsonisation | natural killer cell | antigen | serum sickness | epitope |

| hypersensitivity | vertical transmission | hyperaemia | interferon | Arthus reaction | aids | anaphylaxis |

| splenomegaly | bacteraemia | humerol | urticaria | allergy | pyrexia | Hodgekins disease | pathogen |

| desensitisation | autoimmunity | lysosyme |

Clues across

23 Term used to describe an allergy that can affect any part of the body (6)

26 Type of protein released by host cells on exposure to infectious agents (10)

29 Part of the antigen to which an antibody attaches; antigenic determinant (7)

31 Part of an antigen to which an antibody attaches (7)

32 Capacity for antibodies and complement components to mark pathogens for phagocytic destruction (12)

34 Type III hypersensitivity reaction caused by exposure to antiserum or medicinal proteins (5, 8)

38 Transmission of a pathogen from mother to foetus or baby during pregnancy or birth (8, 12)

41 Sign of allergic reaction characterized by itchy red welts; hives (9)

42 Presence of viable bacteria in the blood (11)

44 Vascular changes associated with localized inflammation (10)

45 Condition commonly caused by infection with the bacterium *Clostridium perfringens* (3, 8)

46 Misdirected response by antibodies and T-lymphocytes against self-antigens (12)

47 Enlargement of the spleen commonly caused by infection (12)

48 Antimicrobial enzyme that occurs in tears and other natural secretions (8)

Clues down

22 Class of immune response that involves secreted antibodies circulating in bodily fluids (7)

24 Abnormal elevation of body temperature; fever (7)

25 Type of lymphoma characterized by abnormal development of B-lymphocytes (9, 7)

27 Damaging immune response by the body to a substance, especially to which it has become hypersensitive (7)

28 Serious or life-threatening reaction to an allergen that may be rapid in onset (11)

30 Lymphocyte capable of binding to certain tumour cells and virus-infected cells without the stimulation of antigens (7, 6, 4)

33 Chronic, potentially life-threatening condition caused by the human immunodeficiency virus (4)

35 Exaggerated immune response resulting from mild antigen exposure (16)

36 Severe, local immune reaction to the injection of an antigen in a sensitized host (6, 8)

37 Non-specific or natural immune system (6)

39 Any substance capable of inducing antibody production (7)

40 Microbial agent capable of causing disease (8)

43 Measure of pathogenicity; the ability of a microorganism to cause disease (9)

ANSWERS

TRUE OR FALSE?

1 **Disorders of the immune system fall into three main categories.**

The three types of immune disorders are:

I. *autoimmune disorders* – when the body initiates an immune response on itself (as in rheumatoid arthritis);

II. *hypersensitivity disorders* – when an allergen enters the body and causes an over-sensitive immune reaction, which may be instant or delayed;

III. *immunodeficiency disorders* – resulting from a suppressed or deficient immune system (such as AIDS, chronic fatigue syndrome (ME) or during cancer treatment).

2 **Inflammation is classified in three main ways** ✗

Inflammation is classified in *two* main ways – it can be either acute or chronic.

I. *acute inflammation* – is part of the body's normal immune response and healing process; it usually occurs for a short duration and resolves quickly (usually 1–2 weeks), after which the body reverts back to its state before the illness or injury;

II. *chronic inflammation* – when the body's immune system attacks healthy cells; it is often linked with autoimmune disorders and occurs when the inflammation does not end, even when the illness or injury has cleared.

3 **An organism that causes an infection in the human body by evading the immune system is called a pathogen.** ✓

A pathogen is defined as a microorganism that causes disease when it enters the human body and avoids the body's immune responses. Pathogens can be transmitted in a variety of ways, depending on the type.

4 | **For infection control, nurses should always wear gloves during patient contact.** ✗

It is not always necessary to wear gloves during patient contact; sometimes they can actually be a mode of transmission for infection. The most effective infection control measure is a good handwashing technique.

5 | **Bacteria contain carbohydrates that may cause infection.** ✗

Pathogenic bacteria contain two different types of *proteins* that cause infection: (1) exotoxins – released during growth; and (2) endotoxins – released when the bacterial cell wall breaks down. Endotoxins cause fevers and do not respond to antibiotics.

6 | **Fungi can be classified as yeasts or moulds.** ✓

Fungi are relatively large compared to other microorganisms. Yeasts are round, single-cell organisms that can survive with or without oxygen. Moulds are filament-like organisms that require oxygen. As part of its natural flora, the body has a range of fungi. However, sometimes they can overproduce, especially when the normal flora becomes unbalanced. Yeast infections sometimes occur during certain antibiotic treatments because the antibiotic will also attack the normal flora in addition to its bacterial target. Most fungal infections (such as athlete's foot) are relatively minor unless the immune system is already compromised (for example, during cancer treatment) or if the infection spreads systemically.

7 | **Parasitic infections are very common in cold climates.** ✗

Infections caused by parasites are *less* common in cold climates but can be very prevalent in hot, moist climates. Most parasitic infections (such as tapeworms) occur in the gastrointestinal (GI) tract. Parasites depend on their host for food and a protective environment, often to the detriment of the host's wellbeing.

8 | **B-cells are responsible for humoral immunity.** ✓

B-cells trigger the humoral (antibody)-mediated immune response. B-cells originate in the bone marrow and mature to become plasma cells that produce antibodies. Antibodies provide immunity by destroying bacteria and viruses before they enter host cells.

MULTIPLE CHOICE

Correct answers identified in **bold italics**

9 **Which of the following is *not* a sign of inflammation?**

a) Heat   **b)** ***Improvement or gain of function***
c) pain   d) redness

Inflammation is part of the innate (non-specific) immune system's response to protect the body from infection, injury or disease. There are five cardinal signs of inflammation: heat, pain, redness, swelling and loss of function. They may differ depending on the location that is affected by inflammation. Inflammation triggers vasodilation, which brings more blood to the affected area. This generates heat and redness because of the increased blood flow in the local area. Cytokines are released into the blood, which increases vascular permeability leading tò localized swelling (oedema) due to the accumulation of fluid in the tissues. The additional fluid can trigger pain due to the inflammatory chemicals stimulating nociceptors, making the affected region more sensitive to pain. Loss of function can occur due to inflammation – for example, a broken bone in the hand may lead to reduced mobility of the hand; this is a protective mechanism of inflammation to allow damaged tissue (in this example, the bone) time to heal and repair.

10 **Tonsillitis is most commonly caused by:**

a) ***viruses***   b) bacteria   c) fungi   d) protozoa

Tonsillitis is an infection most commonly caused by a virus, often those that frequently affect the respiratory system (such as the influenza virus), but it can also be caused by bacteria. Irrespective of the cause, the main symptom is a sore throat, often accompanied by red, swollen tonsils, which may have visible pus-filled spots. As a result, the patient may have difficulty swallowing. The patient may also present with a headache, coughing, fatigue, pain in the ears or neck. If the tonsillitis is caused by a virus, there may be associated flu-like symptoms. If it is bacterial, the face may be flushed or have a rash. Most GPs will diagnose tonsillitis based on the symptoms, however, a throat swab may be taken if bacterial infection is suspected and in patients who are immune-compromised or where the infection is recurrent. For an isolated episode, the infection usually subsides within a few days and painkillers may be prescribed to ease symptoms. If the infection is known to be bacterial, an antibiotic may be prescribed to treat the infection. For recurrent infections, surgical removal of the tonsils (tonsillectomy) may be recommended.

11 **Pathogens can be transmitted via which of the following routes?**

a) airborne

b) arthropods

c) direct and indirect contact

d) all of the above

When the body's first-line defence mechanisms are overcome by a pathogen, infection can occur. Pathogens can enter the body through the GI tract, the respiratory tract or through the skin. Transmission may be airborne or through direct or indirect contact with skin bodily fluids or a solid surface; pathogens may also be spread by arthropods (such as flies, lice, mites).

12 **Which of the following is a major protein cascade that supports the inflammatory response?**

a) inflammation system

b) complimentary system

c) complement system

d) compliment system

The proteins of the complement system continuously circulate in the blood but are usually inactive. When the antigen of a pathogen is encountered by an antibody in the body, the proteins of the complement cascade become activated to initiate and support the inflammatory response. The complement cascade enhances the inflammatory response in two ways: (1) by increasing vascular permeability and (2) promoting chemotaxis (movement of white blood cells to the area of inflammation). It also supports the immune response by encouraging phagocytosis of the foreign bodies and helping breakdown of the foreign cell (cytolysis). (*Hint*: to distinguish the spelling, think complement – with an E – <u>e</u>nhances the inflammatory response).

FILL IN THE BLANKS

13 *Infection* **can occur when a pathogen or disease-causing substance enters the body.**

Infection results when the tissue-destroying microorganisms enter the body and multiply. Infections can result in a minor illness (for example, the common cold) but sometimes can induce more life-threatening conditions, such as septicaemia (blood poisoning). Septicaemia causes vasodilation and multiple organ dysfunction throughout the body.

14 *Viral* **infections can occur when normal immune and inflammatory responses fail.**

Viruses are intracellular parasites that contain genetic material but need a specific host cell to replicate inside. The virus replicates in the host cell using the host cell's DNA. It remains there undetected by the immune system until it is released and infects other cells.

15 *Opportunistic* **infections usually occur in people with weakened immune systems.**

When the immune system is weakened or compromised, this presents an 'opportunity' for pathogens to infect the body. Situations when the immune system may be weakened include therapeutic immunosuppression (following organ transplant), cancer treatment, antibiotic treatment as a result of malnutrition, acquired immunodeficiency syndrome (AIDS) and pregnancy.

16 **In the cell-mediated immune response,** *T*-**cells respond directly to the foreign antigen.**

T-cells respond directly to antigens on the cell surface of invading pathogens. Their response triggers the secretion of lymph proteins (called lymphokines), which destroy target cells such as virus-infected or cancer cells. T-cells can be classified as helper, killer or suppressor cells. Helper T-cells stimulate B-cells to mature into plasma cells, which synthesize and secrete antibodies. Killer (or cytotoxic) T-cells bind to the cell surface of the invading pathogen and destroy them. Suppressor T-cells reduce the humoral-mediated immune response.

MATCH THE TERMS

| 17 | Anaphylaxis   **B. hypersensitivity**

Anaphylaxis is an acute allergic reaction triggered by exposure to an antigen. Symptoms include sudden onset and rapid progression of urticaria (hives) and respiratory distress. A severe reaction can also cause vascular collapse, systemic shock and even death.

- *Causes*: There are many possible triggering antigens, including vaccine serums, hormones, certain enzymes, anaesthetics, latex, foods, blood/blood products or sensitizing drugs, the most common of which is penicillin.

- *Pathophysiology*: Upon first exposure to the allergen, the immune system becomes sensitized to the allergen and produces specific antibodies (called immunoglobulin E, IgE) that remain on the surface of mast cells. In a second exposure to the allergen, the IgE molecules bind to the allergen and sensitize mast cells, which degranulate and release histamine (and other inflammatory mediators). Histamine causes constriction of some smooth muscle, resulting in vasodilation and increased vascular permeability (Figure 2.1). In an anaphylactic reaction vasodilation is very rapid, which causes a sudden drop in blood pressure; this is accompanied by contraction of smooth muscle in the respiratory airways, which may result in wheezing and dyspnoea.

- *Signs and symptoms*: Immediately after exposure, patients may report a feeling of severe anxiety. This is accompanied by dyspnoea (shortness of breath), weakness, sweating and urticaria.

- *Diagnosis and treatment:* Take the patient's history; note signs and symptoms; monitor heart rate, respiratory rate and blood pressure. An injection of adrenaline (epinephrine) should be given, followed by massage of the injection site to improve the drug distribution in the circulation; if the patient is unconscious, it can be administered by intravenous (IV) injection.

Figure 2.1 The mechanism of anaphylaxis

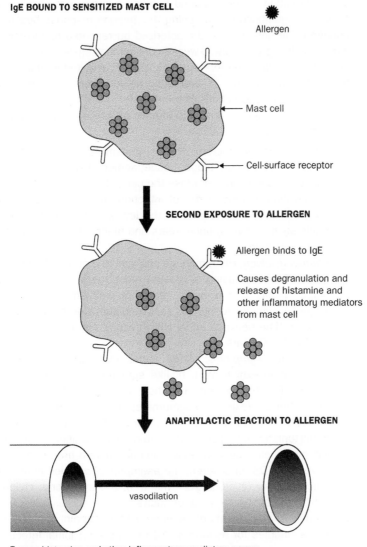

IgE BOUND TO SENSITIZED MAST CELL

Allergen

Mast cell

Cell-surface receptor

SECOND EXPOSURE TO ALLERGEN

Allergen binds to IgE

Causes degranulation and release of histamine and other inflammatory mediators from mast cell

ANAPHYLACTIC REACTION TO ALLERGEN

vasodilation

Excess histamine and other inflammatory mediators cause:
• smooth muscle contraction, resulting in bronchoconstriction;
• vasodilation, which triggers a sudden decrease in blood pressure;
• increased vascular permeability causing oedema and the appearance of hives.

18 HIV disease **C. immunodeficiency**

Infection with human immunodeficiency virus (HIV) causes a progressive destruction of the acquired immune system, specifically the T-cells (T4 lymphocytes), meaning the immune response becomes impaired. The infection is characterized by repeated opportunistic infections that progressively weaken the immune system by destroying helper T-cells, therefore suppressing the acquired immune system. When the number of circulating helper T-cells becomes very low, opportunistic infections present a significant threat of serious disease. The patient is now said to have developed acquired immunodeficiency syndrome (AIDS).

- *Causes and risk factors*: HIV is transmitted in body fluids. Contact with infected blood, tissue, semen or vaginal fluids can cause infection. HIV can cross the placenta and infect a foetus; the newborn is also at risk of infection during delivery and via breast milk. It is thought that the levels of HIV in other body fluids such as saliva, urine, tears and faeces are insufficient to cause infection.

- *Pathophysiology*: HIV requires a host cell to replicate. It destroys helper T-cells, causing a gradual reduction in the number of helper T-cells in the body, therefore weakening the body's acquired immune responses (cell-mediated and humoral). The average time between initial HIV infection and development of AIDS is 8–10 years.

- *Signs and symptoms:* After initial exposure, an infected person may exhibit mild, flu-like symptoms or no symptoms at all. After this primary infection, an individual may remain asymptomatic (exhibit no symptoms) for up to 10 years. As the disease progresses, an infected individual may begin to exhibit opportunistic infections. Repeated opportunistic infections will overwhelm the weakened immune system and the patient develops AIDS. In children, the asymptomatic period is usually much shorter (averaging 17 months); the symptoms children exhibit are similar to those of adults.

- *Diagnosis and treatment*: A person may remain negative for HIV antibodies for as long as 14 months after initial infection, although a positive test for HIV antibodies is usually obtained 3–7 weeks post-exposure. Antibody tests in neonates can be unreliable due to the presence of maternal antibodies in the child for up to 18 months after birth – this can lead to false-positive results in neonatal tests. Routine blood tests monitor

ANSWERS

helper T-cell count and HIV viral load in the blood, which are used to evaluate the level of immunosuppression. There is no cure for HIV or AIDS but several drugs exist to slow the progression of the disease. Certain antiretroviral drugs (called highly active antiretroviral therapy, HAART treatment) reduce replication of the virus and hence slow HIV progression. Anti-infective drugs can also be prescribed to limit the number of opportunistic infections that will progressively weaken the immune system. Anti-neoplastic agents can be used to treat the rare cancers often associated with HIV and AIDS.

19 | Rheumatoid arthritis   **A. autoimmune**

A chronic, systemic, inflammatory autoimmune disorder causing destruction of the peripheral joints and surrounding muscles, tendons, ligaments and blood vessels. Rheumatoid arthritis patients can undergo spontaneous remission but also unpredictable exacerbation of their condition. It is more prevalent in females than males and usually affects patients between the ages of 20 and 50.

- *Causes and risk factors*: The cause remains unknown but genetic influences, hormones and infections are thought to be involved. Viruses are thought to trigger rheumatoid arthritis in people who have a genetic susceptibility for the disease.
- *Pathophysiology*: Exposure to an antigen triggers the formation of altered antibodies that the body does not recognize as its own. Since they are recognized as foreign, the body then forms another antibody against them, called rheumatoid factor, which causes inflammation. This inflammation eventually results in cartilage damage. The continued immune response includes activation of the complement cascade, which stimulates release of inflammatory mediators thus exacerbating joint destruction.
- *Signs and symptoms:* Initially symptoms are non-specific, and include fatigue, malaise, weight loss and persistent low-grade fever. As the inflammation progresses, more specific symptoms are observed such as swelling around the joint that may be warm and/or painful. These symptoms occur particularly in the fingers, but also in wrists, elbows, knees and ankles.
- *Diagnosis and treatment:* No test will provide a definitive diagnosis of rheumatoid arthritis but there are useful indicative tests:
  - X-ray – soft-tissue swelling and bone demineralization are observable and X-rays can be used to determine the extent of cartilage and bone destruction.

□ Testing for presence of rheumatoid factor – although this is not sufficient to diagnose the disease, it is useful in determining prognosis. The prognosis worsens as nodules and vasculitis (inflammation of blood or lymph vessels) develop.

Since it is a chronic illness, rheumatoid arthritis usually requires lifelong treatment and sometimes surgery on joints that are painful or damaged. Treatments to reduce pain and inflammation help to maintain quality of life. Nonsteroidal anti-inflammatory drugs (NSAIDs) are the main type of painkiller used since they decrease inflammation and relieve joint pain. Immunosuppressants are sometimes used early in the disease to halt its progression. Tumour necrosis factor (TNF) alpha-blockers are a relatively new class of drug that are proving effective in treating adults and children with rheumatoid arthritis and other autoimmune disorders. Patients are also encouraged to practise certain exercises to maintain joint function.

| 20 | Lupus erythematosus | **A. autoimmune** |

A chronic, inflammatory, autoimmune disorder affecting the connective tissues. There are two forms of lupus erythematosus: systemic and discoid. Systemic lupus erythematosus (SLE) affects multiple organs and can be fatal. It is the more common form of the condition. It is seen more often in females, particularly those of Afro-Caribbean origin. Discoid lupus erythematosus only affects the skin.

- *Causes*: The exact cause of SLE is unknown. It is thought to be a combination of genetic and environmental factors. Possible triggers include viruses, infection, stress, prolonged use of medication, sunlight exposure, hormones and endocrine changes (including puberty, menopause and childbirth).

- *Pathophysiology*: The body produces antibodies against its own cells, which suppress its normal immune responses. A feature of SLE is that patients produce antibodies against many different types of its own tissues such as red blood cells, white blood cells, platelets and even its own organs.

- *Signs and symptoms*: Symptoms of lupus can vary. Some people only experience a mild form of the condition, whereas others are more severely affected and may develop serious complications. As with other autoimmune disorders, there are no specific symptoms. SLE primarily causes fatigue, joint pain and skin rashes (particularly the 'butterfly rash' over the cheeks and bridge of the nose), as the immune system attacks the body's tissue and cells. Certain blood disorders may be detected such as anaemia, leukopenia, lymphopenia and thrombocytopenia. An elevated erythrocyte sedimentation rate (ESR) may also occur.

- *Diagnosis and treatment*: SLE can be difficult to diagnose because symptoms vary between patients. Active disease is diagnosed by decreased serum complement levels, since complement levels decrease during active SLE episodes.

Drugs are the main form of treatment for SLE. In mild conditions, NSAIDs are sufficient to control the arthritis and joint pain. Topical corticosteroids can be applied to treat skin lesions. Hydroxychloroquine (normally used to treat malaria) is also effective in treating some symptoms of SLE, such as skin rashes, joint and muscle pain and fatigue, although there can be complications associated with this type of medication. Patients are also advised to protect themselves from the sun.

21 Allergic rhinitis   **B. hypersensitivity**

When airborne allergens are inhaled, they may trigger an immune response in the upper airway, which may cause inflammation of the nasal mucous membranes (rhinitis) or conjunctivitis (inflammation of the membrane lining inside the eyelids and covering the eyeball). Seasonal allergic rhinitis is commonly known as hay fever.

- *Causes*: The airborne allergens that trigger the disorder include dust, animal fibres, pollen (triggers hay fever) or work-related allergens (such as flour, chemical vapours or latex).
- *Pathophysiology*: Allergic rhinitis is a hypersensitivity response to an environmental allergen. The nasal and mucous membranes swell and may lead to secondary sinus or middle ear infections. Complications include pneumonia and bronchitis.
- *Signs and symptoms*: Allergic rhinitis can cause cold-like symptoms, such as sneezing and runny nose; patients may also experience headache or sinus pain and have an itchy throat. Dark circles may develop under the eyes as a result of venous congestion in the maxillary sinuses.
- *Diagnosis and treatment*: Analysis of nasal secretions may show elevated levels of the white blood cells. The best advice for any allergy involves controlling symptoms and avoiding allergens known to trigger infection. Antihistamines are the main type of drug prescribed to reduce the runny nose and watery eyes symptoms. However, some antihistamines can have undesired sedative effects, although non-sedating antihistamines are also available.

PUZZLE GRID

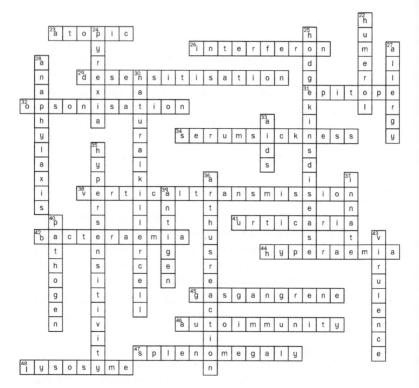

23 atopic
26 interferon
22 humeral (down)
25 hodgkin (down)
27 allergy (down)
28 anaphylaxis (down)
29 desensitisation
24 pyraxauralkapsill (down)
31 epitope
32 opsonisation
30 naturalkiller (down)
33 addison (down)
34 serumsickness
35 hypspsstitivt (down)
36 authurose (down)
37 innate (down)
38 verticaltransmission
40 p (down)
41 urticaria
42 bacteraemia
44 hyperaemia
43 virulence (down)
45 gasgangrene
46 autoimmunity
47 splenomegaly
48 lysosyme

3 The nervous system and special senses

INTRODUCTION

The nervous system is made up of the central and peripheral nervous systems. Together they work to receive, integrate and initiate response to stimuli from inside and outside the body.

Nervous system disorders may be acute or chronic. Many acute conditions can be life-threatening if not diagnosed and treated quickly. Chronic disorders of the nervous system, such as Huntington's disease, are frequently irreversible and life-limiting.

Neurological assessment skills are essential in nursing, particularly assessment of consciousness using the Glasgow Coma Scale (GCS). This scale measures how severely damaged the brain is based on a patient's verbal responses, physical reflexes and how easily they can open their eyes. The highest score is 15, meaning a patient knows where they are and can speak and move as instructed.

With chronic, life-limiting neurological disorders, patients are normally prescribed neuroprotective drugs that slow neurodegeneration. Alongside drug therapy, these patients require social support to help them maintain good quality of life and independence for as long as possible.

Nurses should appreciate how nervous system disorders can have serious and sometimes devastating and degenerative consequences for many organ systems because of its pivotal role in providing communication between the body's organs and systems.

Useful resources

Nurses! Test Yourself in Anatomy and Physiology (2nd edition)
Chapter 3

Ross and Wilson's Anatomy and Physiology in Health and Illness (14th edition)
Chapters 7 and 8

Symptoms, Diagnosis and Treatment (1st edition)
Chapters 2 and 3

TRUE OR FALSE?

Are the following statements true or false?

1 The most common cause of problems with the sensory organs is an inability to detect stimuli.

2 Induced hypertension is neuroprotective.

3 In demyelinating conditions, neural conduction rates are often increased.

4 Hypothermia is neuroprotective because it reduces cerebral oxygen demand.

5 Elevated serum glucose is neuroprotective.

6 A red rash that disappears when a glass is applied is a simple diagnostic test for meningitis.

7 Epilepsy is triggered by abnormal electrical stimulation of neurones in the brain.

8 Stroke occurs when the circulation to the heart is suddenly impaired.

9 Multiple sclerosis is caused by progressive demyelination of the axons of neurones.

10 Alzheimer's disease is a progressive, degenerative disorder of the cerebrospinal fluid.

11 Guillain-Barré syndrome is caused by demyelination of central nerves.

12 Multiple sclerosis patients frequently report the same two initial symptoms.

13 Myasthenia gravis is a neurodegenerative condition character-ized by involuntary tremors, progressive muscle rigidity and loss of movement.

MULTIPLE CHOICE

Identify one correct answer for each of the following:

14 A head trauma can cause what type of eye injury?

a) retinal detachment

b) cataract

c) glaucoma

d) macular degeneration

15 Which of the following is the most common cause of a perforated eardrum?

a) changes in air pressure

b) middle ear infections

c) loud noise

d) mechanical injury

16 Which of the following is considered a stroke warning?

a) chronic obstructive pulmonary disorder

b) deep-vein thrombosis

c) myocardial infarction

d) transient ischaemic attack

17 Which acronym has been introduced and publicized to increase recognition of stroke signs and symptoms?

a) BACK

b) FACE

c) FAST

d) SLOW

18 Meningitis causes inflammation of which part of the brain and spinal cord?

a) white matter

b) neurones

c) grey matter

d) meninges

19 The main treatment for bacterial meningitis is usually:

a) no drugs, just rest and fluids

b) paracetamol, rest and fluids

c) antibiotics, rest and fluids

d) antihistamines, rest and fluids

20 The main symptoms of Parkinson's disease are:

a) sensory symptoms

b) motor symptoms

c) dementia symptoms

d) immunological symptoms

21 Treatment for Parkinson's disease is mainly aimed at:

a) reversing symptoms

b) relieving symptoms

c) stimulating dopamine production

d) stimulating motor cortex

22 Which of the following tests is *not* used to diagnose Guillain-Barré syndrome?

a) an electrocardiogram

b) analysis of protein levels in the cerebrospinal fluid

c) electrophysiology studies

d) electromyography

23 The most useful tool for diagnosing multiple sclerosis is:

a) a CT scan

b) an MRI scan

c) blood tests

d) an electroencephalogram

24 Cerebrospinal fluid helps maintain constant:

a) arterial blood pressure

b) venous blood pressure

c) intracranial pressure

d) thoracic pressure

FILL IN THE BLANKS

Fill in the blanks in each statement using the options in this box.
Not all of them are required, so choose carefully!

Huntington's	lumbar puncture	Fragile X
brain	Guillain-Barré	Parkinson's
vertigo	symptoms	ultrasound
clot-busting	dysaesthesia	complications

25 A _____ _____ detects elevated pressure in cerebrospinal fluid.

26 A _____ scan is used to confirm diagnosis of a stroke.

27 When an ischaemic stroke is quickly diagnosed, patients can be treated with _____-_____ drugs.

28 The main symptom of _____-_____ syndrome is progressive ascending muscle weakness and paralysis.

29 A diagnosis of _____ disease is based on the patient's age, history and signs/symptoms rather than laboratory tests.

30 _____ disease is an incurable, inherited disease that causes gradual deterioration and loss of brain function.

31 _____ describes an inappropriate sense of motion.

32 Headache, muscle weakness and paraesthesia are _____ that are common to many nervous system disorders.

PUZZLE GRID

Use the word bank (below) and clues to solve the puzzle.

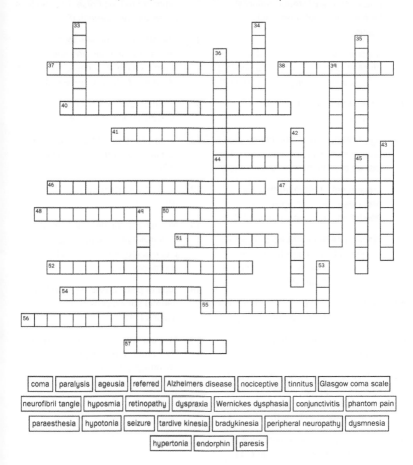

Word bank:

coma | paralysis | ageusia | referred | Alzheimers disease | nociceptive | tinnitus | Glasgow coma scale

neurofibril tangle | hyposmia | retinopathy | dyspraxia | Wernickes dysphasia | conjunctivitis | phantom pain

paraesthesia | hypotonia | seizure | tardive kinesia | bradykinesia | peripheral neuropathy | dysmnesia

hypertonia | endorphin | paresis

Clues across

37 Progressive neurologic disorder commonly associated with loss of memory and cognitive function (10, 7)

38 Decrease in muscle tone (9)

Clues down

33 Sudden, uncontrolled electrical disturbance in the brain; common symptom of epilepsy (7)

34 Weakened or impaired muscle movement; partial paralysis (7)

Clues across (continued)

40 Impaired comprehension of speech and language often resulting from trauma to the posterior temporal lobe of the brain's dominant hemisphere (9, 9)

41 Abnormal sensation of the skin (tingling, pricking, burning numbness) with no apparent physical cause (12)

44 Loss of taste functions of the tongue (7)

46 Aggregates of phosphorylated tau protein commonly accepted as a bio-marker of Alzheimer's disease (11, 6)

47 Impairment of memory that can occur as a discrete episode or persist as a chronic condition (9)

48 Pituitary peptide that acts on opiate receptors to increase feelings of pleasure and wellbeing, and reduce perception of pain (9)

50 Inflammation or infection of the outer membrane of the eye; pink eye (14)

51 Reduction in the ability to detect odours (8)

52 Objective scale used to describe the extent of impaired consciousness in all types of acute medical and trauma patients (7, 4, 5)

54 Proliferative or non-proliferative vascular disease of the eye (11)

55 Excessive muscle tone causing reduced joint mobility or contracture (10)

56 Post-amputation phenomena in which painful sensations continue to be perceived in the trauma region (7, 4)

57 Type of pain perceived at a location other than the site of stimulus (8)

Clues down (continued)

35 Perception of noise which has no external source; associated with exposure to loud noise, hearing loss or certain medications (8)

36 Damage to the nerves located outside of the brain and spinal cord, often causing weakness, numbness and pain, in the extremities (10, 10)

39 Common side effect of antipsychotic medications (7, 7)

42 Slowness of movement; cardinal symptom of Parkinson's disease (12)

43 Loss of voluntary muscle function (9)

45 Neurological disorder that impacts an individual's ability to plan and process motor tasks; developmental coordination disorder (9)

49 Type of pain caused by potentially harmful stimuli causing damage to tissues (11)

53 Medical emergency characterized by a state of prolonged unconsciousness (4)

ANSWERS

TRUE OR FALSE?

1 **The most common cause of problems with the sensory organs is an inability to detect stimuli.**

There are three possible problems that can account for disorders of the sensory organs (eyes, ears, nose, tongue and sensory receptors for touch, pressure or temperature):

I. stimuli cannot be detected by receptors;
II. receptors do not respond normally to stimuli;
III. integration and communication pathways are defective.

Detection of stimuli is the main problem associated with sensory disorders; examples include cataracts on the eyes, which prevent light from reaching the retina of the eye and conductive deafness, where sound is unable to enter the inner ear. Examples of sensory disorders where stimuli reach receptors but receptors do not respond normally include colour blindness, inherited deafness and deafness caused by loud noise. Examples of disorders caused by defects in integration and communication of stimuli include glaucoma or brain damage caused by stroke or other cranial trauma.

2 **Induced hypertension is neuroprotective.**

This is part of controlled triple 'H' therapy: hypertension to increase perfusion; haemodilution to increase plasma volume and pressure; and hypervolaemia to do both. This procedure can be used to treat vasospasm (a serious complication of subarachnoid haemorrhage (SAH)); its aim is to keep the blood vessels open (haemodilution and hypervolaemia) and the tissue perfused (hypertension), to prevent ischaemia in the brain.

3 **In demyelinating conditions, neural conduction rates are often increased.**

In demyelinating conditions, the myelin covering on the axon of the neurone is depleted or reduced. Thinner myelin allows sodium channels to spread out from the nodes, thus slowing conduction rates of the electrical nerve impulse, and saltatory conduction is lost. The most common demyelinating condition is multiple sclerosis (MS). Others include diphtheria, which is caused by a bacterial infection of the respiratory tract and Guillain-Barré syndrome, which can occur after a viral infection (see Answer 11).

4 **Hypothermia is neuroprotective because it reduces cerebral oxygen demand.** ✔

There is a 50% reduction in oxygen demand as core body temperature falls from 37°C to 27°C; this happens because hypothermia slows the metabolism (which requires oxygen), therefore reducing the risk of ischaemic tissue injury, hence protecting the delicate nervous tissue. This is why transplant organs are stored in ice and it is the basis for therapeutic (induced) hypothermia where the patient's body temperature is reduced under medical supervision. Some brain injury patients have a better long-term outcome after this treatment.

5 **Elevated serum glucose is neuroprotective.** ✘

Elevated levels of plasma glucose (hyperglycaemia) are considered dangerous. They cause a greater-than-expected fall in intracellular pH because excess glucose may produce lactic acid (which lowers blood pH) during ischaemia. Furthermore, glucose-induced arteriolar dilation impairs effective vasoregulation and facilitates hypertensive damage to all organs.

6 **A red rash that disappears when a glass is applied is a simple diagnostic test for meningitis.** ✘

The red rash should *not* disappear when a glass is gently pressed on the skin. There are many signs and symptoms of meningitis, including headache, stiff neck, aversion to light, fatigue, vomiting, seizures, fever and chills. Infants and children may be fretful or refuse food. Other diagnostic tests include Brudzinski's sign or Kernig's sign. In Brudzinski's sign, a patient in the dorsal recumbent position (lying on back, head and shoulders) involuntarily flexes the hips and knees when the neck is bent forward. For Kernig's sign, pain or resistance when the hip and knee are flexed in the supine position indicates meningitis.

7 **Epilepsy is triggered by abnormal electrical stimulation of neurones in the brain.** ✔

Neurones in the brain are hyperstimulated, resulting in an excessive amount of electrical activity. This may trigger convulsive movements, of which there are a number of different types. The cerebral cortex is the region of the brain that triggers epileptic seizures. The specific area where the seizure occurs (the epileptogenic focus) varies and is determined by observing the symptoms that occur during a seizure.

8 **Stroke occurs when the circulation to the heart is suddenly impaired.**

Stroke or cerebrovascular accident (CVA) describes a decrease in circulation to the brain. A reduction in circulation to the heart is described as myocardial infarction (MI), or heart attack. CVA can occur when the brain is deprived of oxygenated blood, this can happen in two ways:

I. a blood vessel in the brain becomes blocked by a blood clot, a blockage that is known as an intracranial or cerebral aneurysm, which can lead to an ischaemic stroke; or

II. a blood vessel in the brain bursts (usually because of an aneurysm) causing a haemorrhagic stroke.

Both events result in the brain tissue being deprived of oxygen, causing necrosis (uncontrolled tissue death) from lack of oxygen and accumulation of toxic carbon dioxide. The majority (70–80%) of strokes are ischaemic events.

9 **Multiple sclerosis is caused by progressive demyelination of the axons of neurones.**

Demyelination describes the loss or destruction of the myelin sheath covering some nerve fibres; this results in their impaired function, preventing the normal conduction of the electrical impulses along affected neurones. After myelin is destroyed, a hard plaque of scar tissue forms in its place and disrupts the conduction of nerve impulses. Symptoms of MS are unpredictable and become irreversible as the disease progresses.

10 **Alzheimer's disease is a progressive, degenerative disorder of the cerebrospinal fluid.**

Alzheimer's disease is a disorder of the cerebral cortex. It is progressive and neurodegenerative. It is a form of dementia and accounts for half of all dementia cases. Degeneration (atrophy) is most notable in the frontal lobes but atrophy occurs in all areas of the cortex with clumps of protein (plaques) forming in the brain as nerve cells become damaged. The exact cause of Alzheimer's disease in unknown, although age is the greatest risk factor, with the majority of those affected being over 65 years old. A family history presents only a slightly higher risk, although symptoms may present earlier. People with Down's syndrome have a higher risk of developing Alzheimer's disease. Symptoms vary with the severity and progression of the disease but include forgetfulness, irritability, mood swings, incontinence, delusions and obsessive/repetitive behaviour. Although there is no cure, medication (acetylcholinesterase inhibitors that prevent chemical breakdown in the brain) may be prescribed to slow the progression of the disease. Other treatments include establishing appropriate care and support for patients and their carers.

11 **Guillain-Barré syndrome is caused by demyelination of central nerves.** ✗

Peripheral nerves are demyelinated in Guillain-Barré syndrome, which is sometimes called acute demyelinating polyneuropathy. It is a cell-mediated, autoimmune disorder that is rapidly progressive and potentially fatal, although patients can make a full recovery. Its precise cause is unknown, although it often occurs in patients who have recently had influenza (viral infection) or respiratory disorders. There are three clinical phases associated with the syndrome. The *acute* phase, when symptoms first develop, lasts 1–3 weeks and ends when no further deterioration is observed. The *plateau* phase is the second phase and can last from a few days to 2 weeks. The *recovery* phase lasts longest; it is thought to correspond with remyelination and can last from 4 months to 3 years. Recovery is not always complete and patients often need rehabilitation assistance in the form of occupational therapy and physiotherapy.

12 **Multiple sclerosis patients frequently report the same two initial symptoms.** ✓

Patients often find it difficult to describe symptoms but a patient history often reveals two initial symptoms, namely visual disturbances and other sensory impairments. After these initial events, symptoms vary and depend on the extent of myelin loss, the site of myelin loss, the extent of any remyelination and the quality of nerve transmission at the synapses after remyelination. Other signs and symptoms include fatigue, muscle weakness, paralysis, poor speech, poor gait, urinary and bowel problems.

13 **Myasthenia gravis is a neurodegenerative condition characterized by involuntary tremors, progressive muscle rigidity and loss of movement.**

These symptoms are characteristic of the neurodegenerative disorder, Parkinson's disease (PD), which affects movement. In Parkinson's, there is a reduction in the amount of the neurotransmitter hormone, dopamine, in the basal ganglia of the brain; this reduces stimulation of the motor cortex in the brain. Myasthenia gravis is an autoimmune disorder that produces sporadic, progressive weakness and fatigue of voluntary muscles. It is relatively rare and most commonly affects females under 40 years. Antibodies in the immune system attack and damage the nerve signal reception areas on muscles (post-synaptic neuromuscular junction) preventing communication between nerve and muscle, which results in a loss of effectiveness of the muscle.

MULTIPLE CHOICE

Correct answers identified in **bold italics**

14 **A head trauma can cause what type of eye injury?**

a) **retinal detachment**   b) cataract
c) glaucoma   d) macular degeneration

A serious head injury can cause the retina to separate from the inner wall of the eye. The most common symptom of retinal detachment is a shadow or 'black curtain' spreading across the vision. Vision may become cloudy as small blood vessels bleed into the vitreous humour of the eye. Symptoms also include floaters in the vision or flashing bright lights. There is no pain with retinal detachment. Risk factors include short-sightedness (because the retina can be thinner) and diabetes. It can occur as a complication of cataract surgery. Surgery to reattach the retina is the only treatment, without which blindness will develop.

Glaucoma is a disease in which the optic nerve is damaged, leading to progressive, irreversible loss of vision. It is often, but not always, associated with increased pressure of the fluid in the eye. Macular degeneration refers to loss of central vision due to denegation of the retina and is the major cause of visual impairment in older adults. Cataracts occur when parts of the lens become cloudy as changes occur in the proteins within the lens. Cataracts reduce the amount of light entering the eye and so vision appears cloudy. They can develop as a complication of diabetes mellitus.

15 **Which of the following is the most common cause of a perforated eardrum?**

a) changes in air pressure   ***b) middle ear infections***
c) loud noise   d) mechanical injury

Although all of the above can cause perforation of the eardrum (tympanic membrane), the most common cause is due to infections of the middle ear. During an ear infection, pus can build up inside the ear, putting pressure on the eardrum. With accumulating pressure the eardrum ruptures, allowing the pus to escape. This mucus discharge is a common symptom of a perforated eardrum. A perforated eardrum can sometimes be caused by injury (such as with a cotton bud) or by shock waves from a very loud noise (such as an explosion). Damage from loud noise often causes severe hearing loss and ringing in the ears (tinnitus). Sudden changes in air pressure, such as changes in altitude in an aircraft, often cause pain in the ear. Occasionally, these sudden pressure changes can perforate the eardrum. This occurs because there is a big difference between the air pressure outside the ear and the air pressure inside the middle ear. A perforated eardrum will often heal by itself within 6–8 weeks. Painkillers may be prescribed to ease symptoms and antibiotics may be administered if the ear is infected. If damage is more serious, surgery may be required.

16 **Which of the following is considered a stroke warning?**

a) chronic obstructive pulmonary disorder
b) deep-vein thrombosis
c) myocardial infarction
d) transient ischaemic attack

Transient ischaemic attack (TIA), or 'mini-stroke', is considered a warning of an impending severe stroke. TIA is a temporary interruption of blood blow, usually in the small distal branches of the brain's arteries, which results in lack of oxygen in the brain. TIAs are thought to be due to small micro-emboli that break off from a thrombus and temporarily halt blood flow and hence reduce oxygen supply. They are said to be transient because symptoms disappear in less than 24 hours and normal neurological function returns. The signs and symptoms are usually an indicator of the affected artery and include double vision, unilateral blindness, lack of coordination, numbness, dizziness, and difficulty with speech (FAST symptoms, see Answer 17). Treatment of a TIA aims to prevent a complete stroke by administering aspirin to thin blood or anticoagulants to reduce development of thrombosis. Symptoms lasting longer than 24 hours indicate a 'full' stroke.

17 | **Which acronym has been introduced and publicized to increase recognition of stroke signs and symptoms?**

a) BACK

b) FACE

c) *FAST – meaning: face, arm, speech, time*

d) SLOW

This acronym has been used to raise awareness of stroke symptoms. It indicates the major signs and symptoms of a stroke: facial drooping or paralysis on one side, weakness or paralysis of one or both arms, and distorted speech. When any of these symptoms arise in a patient, people are encouraged to immediately seek emergency medical help. The earlier a patient receives treatment for a stroke, the less severe the long-term neurological effects will be. Patients with suspected ischaemic stroke will be immediately treated with a 'clot-busting' (or thrombolytic) medicine called alteplase, which dissolves blood clots. However, alteplase is only effective if used during the first 3 hours after a stroke has taken place. After an ischaemic stroke, long-term preventative treatment may include aspirin or anticoagulants (such as heparin or warfarin) to thin the blood and reduce the risk of further clots developing. In haemorrhagic stroke patients, emergency surgery on the skull (craniotomy) is often required to remove any blood from the brain and repair any burst blood vessels. Blood pressure- and/or cholesterol-modifying medications may also be necessary long-term treatments after both types of stroke.

18 | **Meningitis causes inflammation of which part of the brain and spinal cord?**

a) white matter

b) neurons

c) grey matter

d) *meninges*

All three membranes of the meninges may be inflamed – dura mater, arachnoid mater and pia mater. The inflammation causes tissues to swell and increases the intracranial pressure (ICP), which reduces blood flow to the brain. Inflammation may be caused by a range of pathogens, but the most common causes of meningitis are bacteria and viruses.

19 **The main treatment for bacterial meningitis is usually:**

a)   no drugs, just rest and fluids
b)   paracetamol, rest and fluids
c)   antibiotics, rest and fluids
d)   antihistamines, rest and fluids

Patients with bacterial meningitis will be treated with IV antibiotics when sent to hospital, followed by oral antibiotics along with rest and plenty of fluids. The most common antibiotic prescribed is penicillin but where there is a known allergy, tetracycline, chloramphenicol or kanamycin can be used instead. For viral meningitis, antibiotics are not appropriate. Until a bacterial cause is excluded, patients will be treated with antibiotics which are then withdrawn upon a viral diagnosis. Patients are advised to rest and remain hydrated.

20 **The main symptoms of Parkinson's disease are:**

a)   sensory symptoms   ***b)   motor symptoms***
c)   dementia symptoms   d)   immunological symptoms

The symptoms of Parkinson's disease (PD) are caused by a decrease in the neurotransmitter dopamine, which affects the motor cortex of the brain, hence the first symptoms that the patient experiences involve motor functions, of which there are four major types. The abbreviation TRAP may be used to describe PD symptoms:

T = tremor;
R = rigidity of muscles – due to joint stiffness;
A = akinesia (slow/impaired muscle movement) or bradykinesia (extremely slow movement);
P = posture instability.

Further symptoms develop including fatigue (due to persistent tremor), dysphagia (difficulty swallowing), impaired speech, increased perspiration, oily skin, insomnia and often depression and mood changes – due to the frustration of the condition. Patients do not suffer from dementia, although it can develop later in the condition. Complications include injury due to falls as a consequence of unstable gait, food aspiration due to impaired swallow, urinary tract infections and skin breakdown due to immobility.

21 **Treatment for Parkinson's disease is aimed at:**

a)   reversing symptoms   ***b)   relieving symptoms***
c)   stimulating dopamine production   d)   stimulating motor cortex

Currently there is no cure for PD or reversal of symptoms. Treatment aims to relieve symptoms and halt progression, maintaining motor function for as long as possible. Drug therapy includes dopamine replacement (but does not stimulate production); however, this can cause adverse effects. Alongside dopamine therapy, patients may receive anticholinergics or antihistamines to reduce tremors. Physiotherapy is also helpful in maintaining muscle function and tone. Deep brain stimulation is a surgical technique to help treat the motor symptoms of PD; a tiny electrical pulse (similar to a heart pacemaker) produces a current in the affected area of the brain, and some PD patients have reported a significant improvement in their motor function. The procedure carries a small risk of stroke and the long-term effectiveness of the procedure has yet to be fully assessed.

22 **Which of the following tests is *not* used to diagnose Guillain-Barré syndrome?**

a) *an electrocardiogram*
b)　analysis of protein levels in the cerebrospinal fluid
c)　electrophysiology studies
d)　electromyography

The tests other than an electrocardiogram (ECG) can be used in the diagnosis of Guillain-Barré syndrome. ECG records the electrical activity of the heart over time by placing electrodes on the surface of the skin. Analysis of cerebrospinal fluid (CSF) may indicate normal white blood cell levels but elevated protein levels and, in severe cases, increased pressure of CSF. The CSF protein levels will continue to increase and peak around 4–6 weeks after the onset of signs and symptoms, indicating widespread inflammation of nerve roots. Electrophysiology studies may indicate slower conduction of electrical impulses between nerves. Electromyography (EMG) records electrical activity produced by the skeletal muscle cells.

23 **The most useful tool for diagnosing multiple sclerosis is:**

a)　a CT scan　　　　　　*b)* *an MRI scan*
c)　blood tests　　　　　　d)　an EEG

Magnetic resonance imaging (MRI) will detect lesions and also indicate the extent of disease. Up to 90% of patients will have detectable lesions by the time an MRI is performed. A CT scan will identify lesions in the brain's white matter. White blood cells (WBC) may be elevated, while an EEG will identify abnormalities in about one-third of patients.

24 **Cerebrospinal fluid helps maintain constant:**

a) arterial blood pressure
b) venous blood pressure
c) intracranial pressure
d) thoracic pressure

Intracranial pressure is affected by brain size and the volumes of intracranial blood and cerebrospinal fluid. Sometimes the effects of raised ICP are more serious than the condition causing it. Raised ICP is usually accompanied by hypertension and bradycardia.

FILL IN THE BLANKS

25 **A *lumbar puncture* detects elevated pressure in cerebrospinal fluid.**

Lumbar puncture (LP or spinal tap) involves inserting a needle into the spinal canal to extract a sample of cerebrospinal fluid (CSF), which is then examined in a laboratory. The CSF may be a cloudy or milky colour, protein levels may be elevated and glucose concentration decreased. Lumbar puncture can be used to diagnose meningitis and a positive Gram stain can assist in identifying the infecting bacteria. A chest X-ray can identify pneumonia, lung abscess or lesions causing fungal meningitis. A CT scan is usually performed before LP to exclude cerebral haemorrhage, haematoma or tumour that may cause meningitis because performing LP on such patients can be dangerous. Lumbar puncture can sometimes be used to administer antibiotics or chemotherapy and, although rare, LP may be used to remove excess CSF and relieve high ICP that can develop in rare conditions such as subarachnoid haemorrhage (SAH) or Lyme disease.

26 **A *brain* scan is used to confirm diagnosis of a stroke.**

All patients with suspected stroke should receive a brain scan within 24 hours. A brain scan will determine the type of stroke (ischaemic or haemorrhagic) and therefore the type of treatment to be given. Some treatments need to be given quickly, so rapid access to diagnostic tests is important. Therefore, if a person is suspected of having a severe stroke, a CT scan is sufficient to identify the region of the stroke and whether it is due to bleeding or a clot. Since a CT scan is much quicker than an MRI scan, the diagnostic time is speeded up, meaning thrombolysis ('clot-busting') treatment can be administered more quickly, which is essential when treating stroke patients. An MRI scan is more appropriate if symptoms are complicated or when the extent or location of the stroke is unclear. The MRI provides more detail of cerebral tissue, allowing smaller strokes to be identified or TIAs in unusual locations.

27 When an ischaemic stroke is quickly diagnosed, patients can be treated with _clot-busting_ drugs.

Ischaemic strokes are caused by clots. Clot-busting (thrombolysis) treatment with alteplase is only effective if administered within a few hours of symptoms developing. The treatment breaks down clots, allowing blood to flow normally. This treatment is not used for patients with haemorrhagic strokes, since it thins the blood and enhances bleeding. Antiplatelet medicines, such as aspirin, reduce the likelihood of future blood clots but again are not advisable as treatment for haemorrhagic strokes. Anticoagulant therapy with heparin or warfarin is recommended for many people with TIA or stroke who have an irregular heart beat (atrial fibrillation) but not for haemorrhagic strokes. Haemorrhagic stroke patients may have emergency cranial surgery (craniotomy) to reduce intracranial pressure and should have blood pressure, blood glucose and oxygen levels monitored. Long-term treatment focuses on lowering blood pressure with angiotensin-converting enzyme (ACE) inhibitor drugs, which widen the blood vessels and reduce blood pressure. Physical and psychological rehabilitation after a serious stroke involves long-term lifestyle changes with many patients developing depression due to their lack of independence after a severe stroke.

28 The main symptom of _Guillain-Barré_ syndrome is progressive ascending muscle weakness and paralysis.

Symptoms of this condition usually arise after an acute infection. Patients begin to notice symmetrical weakness that usually affects the lower limbs first and rapidly progresses, in an ascending fashion, up the legs. Patients generally notice weakness in their legs or legs that tend to buckle, with or without numbness or tingling (dysaesthesia). As the weakness progresses upward, usually over periods of hours to days, the arms and facial muscles also become affected. Patients are often very distressed and seek medical attention at this stage. Patients must be monitored as the paralysis spreads, since it may become life-threatening if it reaches the respiratory or cardiac muscles. Patients are often admitted to intensive care units.

29 **A diagnosis of _Parkinson's_ disease is based on the patient's age, history and signs/symptoms rather than laboratory tests.**

Laboratory tests provide little diagnostic information during investigations for PD. However, a urinalysis test may indicate decreased dopamine levels. A CT or MRI scan may be used to exclude other disorders, such as a tumour, that could cause similar symptoms. Initial diagnosis is usually made based on symptoms, history and clinical examination. If PD is suspected, the patient would be referred to a specialist such as a neurologist or geriatrician.

30 **_Huntington's_ disease is an incurable, inherited disease that causes gradual deterioration and loss of brain function.**

Although rare, Huntington's disease has devastating consequences for the families it affects. The major symptom involves a decline in motor, cognitive and behavioural functions that are usually first observed in early adulthood (between 20 and 35 years old). These progressively decline, leading to dementia and death (although death is usually due to a secondary cause such as heart failure, pneumonia or other infection). As symptoms progress, the patient needs increasing nursing care, particularly in the later stages of the disease. Diagnosis is by genetic testing for the faulty gene, although nowadays families that carry the defective gene would probably be aware of their risk before symptoms develop. No treatment currently exists, and progression cannot be slowed. Speech and occupational therapy are recommended, while many patients will be prescribed medication to control involuntary tremors and some require antidepressants to treat mood swings and depression.

31 **_Vertigo_ describes an inappropriate sense of motion.**

People who experience vertigo report a sensation of movement or spinning even when they are completely still; symptoms also include nausea and loss of balance. It is commonly caused by a problem with the balance mechanisms within the inner ear due to viral infection, although it can also be caused by nerve damage between the middle ear and the brain, or by damage to the brain itself. Initial treatment is with an antihistamine such as cyclizine or prochlorperazine – both will alleviate the nausea associated with vertigo. Patients often find relief from symptoms by lying still in a dark, quiet room. Vertigo that reoccurs or persists may be caused by an underlying condition, such as tinnitus or Ménière's disease, and should be investigated.

32 **Headache, muscle weakness and paraesthesia are _symptoms_ that are common to many nervous system disorders.**

The symptoms of nervous system disorders can be diverse, although headache, muscle weakness and paraesthesia (numbness or tingling) accompany many disorders of this system. Headaches are usually due to muscle tension. Muscle weakness can be caused by muscle diseases (myopathies) or neurological diseases (such as demyelinating diseases), and it is essential that the underlying cause of muscle weakness is determined for accurate diagnosis and treatment. Paraesthesia may be temporary or permanent.

PUZZLE GRID

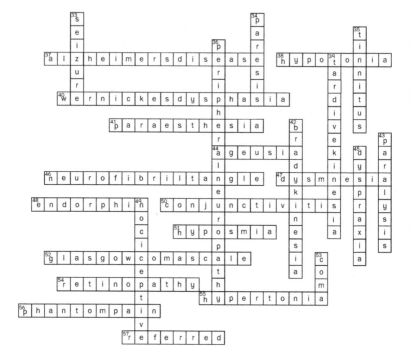

4 The endocrine system

INTRODUCTION

The hypothalamus in the brain is vital for regulating hormones, the chemical messengers of the endocrine system. The other organs of the endocrine system include the adrenal glands, the pancreas, the pituitary gland and the thyroid gland. Feedback systems regulate the endocrine system by controlling the production of hormones.

If a patient has abnormal levels of a hormone circulating in the blood, it may be due to a disorder of the endocrine system caused by abnormal secretion of the hormones, poor response to hormones by their receptor organs or cells, inflammation or a tumour of the hormone-producing gland.

Many endocrine disorders have very general symptoms such as weight loss or gain, fatigue and nausea. Therefore, a detailed patient history and blood tests are usually required to achieve an accurate diagnosis. Patients with an endocrine disorder should be assessed for defects in the gland, problems with the release of hormones, transport of hormones or a problem with the effector organ.

Knowing how the endocrine system is responsible for continuous communication and control can help nurses understand how disruption of this system can lead to widespread disorder in the body.

Useful resources

Nurses! Test Yourself in Anatomy and Physiology (2nd edition)
Chapter 4

Ross and Wilson's Anatomy and Physiology in Health and Illness (14th edition)
Chapter 9

TRUE OR FALSE?

Are the following statements true or false?

| 1 | The aetiology of type 1 diabetes mellitus has been associated with several specific environmental factors.

| 2 | Type 1 diabetes mellitus is insulin-independent.

| 3 | Gestational diabetes mellitus occurs during pregnancy.

| 4 | Diabetes insipidus exists in two forms.

| 5 | Cushing's syndrome is caused by excessive aldosterone secretion by the adrenal cortex.

| 6 | A symptom of hyperthyroidism is decreased weight.

| 7 | Graves' disease is a form of hyperthyroidism.

| 8 | In hypothyroidism, metabolic processes are suppressed.

MULTIPLE CHOICE

Identify one correct answer for each of the following:

9 Which of the following is a symptom of hypoglycaemia?

a) polydipsia

b) dehydration

c) palpitations

d) polyuria

10 The target of glycaemic control is an HbAlc blood level of:

a) < 42 mmol/mol

b) 45 mmol/mol

c) 48 mmol/mol

d) > 53 mmol/mol

11 Diabetes insipidus is caused by a deficiency in:

a) insulin

b) renin

c) angiotensin

d) antidiuretic hormone

12 Which of these disorders is *not* related to the thyroid gland?

a) Addison's disease

b) Graves' disease

c) goitre

d) hyperthyroidism

13 Cushing's syndrome is characterized by an excess of which hormone?

a) antidiuretic hormone

b) glucagon

c) glucocorticoid

d) aldosterone

14 Which of the following is *not* a chronic complication of pheochromocytoma?

a) persistent hypertension

b) glucose intolerance

c) hypermetabolism

d) anhidrosis

15 Which of the following is a symptom of hypothyroidism?

a) diarrhoea

b) constipation

c) sensitivity to cold

d) unexplained weight loss

FILL IN THE BLANKS

Fill in the blanks in each statement using the options in this box.
Not all of them are required, so choose carefully!

Addison's	Cushing's	Parkinson's
hypothyroidism	microvascular	macrovascular
ketoacidosis	glucagon	

16 _____ is recognized as a serious acute complication of diabetes mellitus.

17 A patient with _____ disease would exhibit symptoms that include weight loss, dehydration and a craving for salty food.

18 A complication of _____ disease is hypertension, which can lead to ischaemic heart disease.

19 _____ stimulates hepatic glucose production and release of glucose into the circulation during periods of hypoglycaemia.

20 Blindness, end-stage renal failure and neuropathy are leading complications of diabetic _____ disease.

PUZZLE GRID

Use the clues and word bank to solve the puzzle.

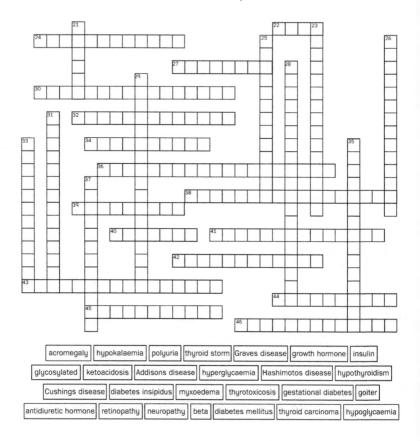

acromegaly | hypokalaemia | polyuria | thyroid storm | Graves disease | growth hormone | insulin

glycosylated | ketoacidosis | Addisons disease | hyperglycaemia | Hashimotos disease | hypothyroidism

Cushings disease | diabetes insipidus | myxoedema | thyrotoxicosis | gestational diabetes | goiter

antidiuretic hormone | retinopathy | neuropathy | beta | diabetes mellitus | thyroid carcinoma | hypoglycaemia

Clues across

22 Cell type found in pancreatic islets that synthesize and secrete insulin and amylin (4)

24 Condition caused by the uncontrolled production of ketone bodies, often resulting from insulin deficiency (12)

Clues down

21 Non-cancerous swelling of the thyroid (6)

23 Adrenal insufficiency associated with low cortisol and aldosterone (8, 7)

Clues across (continued)

27 Excessive urination; frequent symptom of diabetes mellitus and diabetes insipidus (8)

30 Uncontrolled proliferation of thyroid cells associated with hoarseness, dysphagia and nodule formation (7, 9)

32 Peptide hormone that stimulates growth, cell reproduction and cell regeneration; somatotropin (6, 7)

34 Hormonal disorder occurring due to excessive growth hormone production in adulthood (10)

36 Elevated levels of blood glucose occurring during pregnancy, which typically resolves after birth (11, 8)

38 Disease in which the secretion of, or response to, the pituitary hormone vasopressin is impaired, resulting in the production of very large quantities of dilute urine (8, 9)

39 Term used to describe dermatological changes associated with advanced hypothyroidism (9)

40 Pancreatic peptide hormone involved in the metabolic regulation of carbohydrates, fats and protein (7)

41 Clinical effects experienced due to an excess secretion of thyroxine and triiodothyronine (14)

42 Low plasma potassium indicative of excessive aldosterone secretion (12)

43 Chronic disease associated with abnormally high levels of glucose in the blood (8, 8)

44 Complication of diabetes characterized by nerve damage and dysfunction (10)

45 Complication of type I or type II diabetes caused by damage to the light-sensitive tissues of the eye (11)

46 Low blood sugar frequently related to diabetes treatment (13)

Clues down (continued)

25 Immune system disorder resulting in hyperthyroidism (6, 7)

26 Underactive thyroid resulting in reduced aspects of metabolism (14)

28 Short peptide, secreted by the posterior pituitary that promotes water conservation; vasopressin (12, 7)

29 Autoimmune condition affecting the thyroid resulting in impaired metabolism (10, 7)

31 Elevated blood glucose levels usually associated with diabetic conditions (14)

33 Form of haemoglobin used to indicate average blood glucose levels over time (12)

35 Condition caused by excessive pituitary secretion of cortisol (8, 7)

37 Life-threatening condition resulting from sudden excessive release of thyroid hormones (7, 5)

ANSWERS

TRUE OR FALSE?

1 **Type 1 diabetes mellitus has been associated with several environmental factors.**

Several important environmental factors are considered to contribute to the development of type I diabetes mellitus. These include aspects of nutrition, viral infections and exposure to some drugs and chemicals. Bovine serum albumin, a major constituent of cow's milk, has been proposed to trigger the production of beta cell autoantibodies, and nitrosamines may exert toxicity on these insulin-producing cells. Some viral infections may result in autoimmune damage to the pancreatic beta cells. Congenital rubella, Epstein-Barr virus and persistent cytomegalovirus infection are suspect in many cases. Several endocrine disrupting drugs and chemicals, including the antimicrobial pentamidine, the antineoplastic streptozotocin, and the toxic dye precursor alloxan, have been implicated in the disease. However, the mechanisms involved in the disease pathways are not clear.

2 **Type 1 diabetes mellitus is insulin-independent.**

Diabetes mellitus (DM) is a chronic condition characterized by excess glucose in the blood. Insulin is a hormone produced by the pancreas that normally regulates the concentration of glucose in the blood. DM can be caused by either:

- insufficient or no insulin being produced; or
- the body is unable to respond to the insulin it produces.

Irrespective of the cause, the result is the same; the body is unable to use the glucose in the blood for energy, resulting in hyperglycaemia. The two major types of diabetes mellitus are: type 1, which *is* insulin-dependent (previously known as insulin-dependent diabetes mellitus – IDDM) and type 2, which is *not* insulin-dependent (previously known as non-insulin-dependent diabetes mellitus). Type 1 DM is caused by the autoimmune destruction or abnormal function of beta cells, usually due to a genetic defect; this prevents sufficient insulin being produced. It usually develops early in life; hence it was also previously known as juvenile diabetes.

Type 2 DM is much more common, accounting for over 90% of all cases of DM. In type 2 DM, the body's cells become unresponsive to insulin and therefore are unable to utilize the glucose obtained from dietary carbohydrates; in addition, the beta cells may be gradually destroyed over time, which increases insulin resistance in patients. It is strongly associated with obesity and previously occurred more frequently in older individuals. With the increase in obesity in children and young people, more cases of type 2 DM are being diagnosed in the younger population. This will have a serious impact on the long-term care and treatment of DM patients who may live with the disease for many decades and will therefore be more at risk of developing complications associated with DM. Initial clinical symptoms of type 2 DM are usually mild and can often be controlled by diet, exercise and weight loss. However, the longer a person lives with the condition, the more severe their symptoms may become, eventually requiring insulin to control blood glucose levels.

3 | **Gestational diabetes mellitus occurs during pregnancy.**　✔

The third type of DM is gestational diabetes, which only develops during pregnancy and disappears after birth. It is caused by changes to the maternal glucose metabolism during pregnancy. Although the condition may be mild and produce few symptoms in the mother, it presents similar dangers to the foetus as other types of diabetes and often babies have a high birth weight and are more at risk of jaundice. Mothers who are already diabetic need to be monitored very closely during pregnancy to reduce the risk of complications related to their diabetes. Those who develop gestational diabetes are at greater risk of type 2 DM later in life.

4 | **Diabetes insipidus exists in two forms.**　✔

Diabetes insipidus (DI) is a rare form of 'diabetes'. It is characterized by frequent drinking (polydipsia) and excretion of a large volume of urine (polyuria) that is very dilute but does not contain glucose (in contrast to diabetes mellitus). The volume of urine is not reduced when fluid intake is reduced, indicating the kidneys are unable to concentrate urine. DI exists in two forms: neurogenic (central) and nephrogenic (renal). Neurogenic DI is the form most frequently encountered in the clinic and is associated with any form of

ADH insufficiency. Nephrogenic DI is caused by an insensitivity of the renal collecting tubules to ADH and can be genetic in origin or acquired.

5 | **Cushing's syndrome is caused by excessive aldosterone secretion by the adrenal cortex.**
Cushing's syndrome is a relatively uncommon condition that occurs in response to excessive cortisol production and is the most frequent complication of Cushing's disease. Cushing's syndrome exists in two main forms: corticotropin-dependent and corticotropin-independent. The corticotropin-dependent form is the most prevalent and is commonly a result of ACTH-secreting pituitary tumours (80–85% of cases). This form is more frequently diagnosed in women. Corticotropin-independent Cushing's syndrome is less common and is usually caused by an adrenal tumour. Adrenal tumours, as opposed to pituitary tumours, are more common in children.

6 | **A symptom of hyperthyroidism is decreased weight.**
Hyperthyroidism (overactive thyroid) causes an increase in metabolic processes characterized by a decrease in body weight despite an increased appetite. Other signs and symptoms include tremors, palpitations, sweating, diarrhoea, heat intolerance, protrusion of the eyes and an enlarged thyroid gland. Weight gain is a symptom of hypothyroidism due to the slowing down of the metabolism.

7 | **Graves' disease is a form of hyperthyroidism.**
Graves' disease is an autoimmune disorder that causes goitre and is the most common cause of hyperthyroidism. Other causes of hyperthyroidism include thyroid tumours, pituitary tumours and inflammation of the thyroid gland.

8 | **In hypothyroidism, metabolic processes are suppressed.**
Hypothyroidism (underactive thyroid) occurs when levels of thyroid hormones in the blood are low. The slowing down of metabolic processes is caused by the decrease in the levels of the triiodothyronine (T_3) and thyroxine (T_4) hormones that regulate metabolic activity and protein synthesis. The disorder is more common in females and people with Down's syndrome. Primary hypothyroidism indicates a problem with the thyroid gland, while secondary hypothyroidism indicates a failure to stimulate normal thyroid function, such as when the pituitary gland does not secrete enough thyroid-stimulating hormone (TSH).

MULTIPLE CHOICE

Correct answers identified in ***bold italics***

9 **Which of the following is a symptom of hypoglycaemia?**

a) polydipsia

b) dehydration

b) palpitations

d) polyuria

Hypoglycaemia is an acute complication of DM; it indicates a lower than normal level of blood glucose (usually lower than 3.8 mmol/L). As the brain tissue and cells are dependent on a continuous supply of glucose from the blood, if the amount of glucose provided by the blood falls, the brain is one of the first organs to be affected. Patients who become hypoglycaemic may exhibit several signs and symptoms, such as sweating, clamminess, feeling cold, paraesthesia, headache, nausea and vomiting, double vision, slurred speech, irritability, confusion, fatigue, poor coordination (sometimes appearing drunk), seizures and they may even lapse into a coma if the condition is not reversed. If conscious, patients may be treated by rapid glucose administration (such as a high glucose drink).

Polydipsia (increased thirst), polyphagia (increased appetite) and polyuria (frequent urination) are the main symptoms of DM. In type 1 DM, such symptoms can develop quickly (even over a few weeks) but in type 2 DM, symptoms are more subtle and develop over a much longer time.

10 **The target of glycaemic control is an HbA1c blood level of:**

a) < 42 mmol/mol

b) 45 mmol/mol

c) 48 mmol/mol

d) > 53 mmol/mol

Glycaemic control is a medical term referring to the average levels of blood glucose in a DM patient. The long-term complications of DM result from many years of hyperglycaemia, so good glycaemic control indicates the condition is quite stable, which is an important goal for DM patients to reduce the risk of complications. Glucose in the blood binds to haemoglobin, forming glycosylated haemoglobin called HbA1c. The higher the HbA1c level, the more glucose is present in the blood, which is undesirable as it can accelerate development of complications associated with hyperglycaemia. Measuring HbA1c provides an accurate reading of blood glucose levels over the previous 2–3 months. Ideally, consecutive readings should be low, < 48 mmol/mol, although the exact target is set for individual patients based on their symptoms. Control and outcomes of both types 1 and 2 DM may be improved by patients using home glucose meters to regularly monitor their blood glucose levels. However, these meters only measure the amount of glucose in the blood at the specific time of testing.

11 **Diabetes insipidus is caused by a deficiency in:**

a) insulin

b) renin

c) angiotensin

d) *antidiuretic hormone*

Diabetes insipidus (DI) is caused by a lack of antidiuretic hormone (ADH), or vasopressin, production (hyposecretion) or lack of renal response to ADH. Hyposecretion may be caused by damage to the pituitary gland which releases ADH, while a lack of renal response may be due to damage to the kidneys, making them insensitive to ADH. Diabetes insipidus caused by hyposecretion of ADH can be treated with hormone replacement therapy. However, renal DI due to insensitivity to ADH is more difficult to treat.

12 **Which of these disorders is *not* related to the thyroid gland?**

a) *Addison's disease*

b) Graves' disease

c) hypothyroidism

d) goitre

Addison's disease is a disorder of the adrenal glands; it is also known as adrenal hypofunction or adrenal dysfunction. The primary form of Addison's disease originates in the adrenal glands and is characterized by low secretion of the steroid hormones, mineralo-corticoids (mainly aldosterone), glucocorticoids (mainly cortisol) and androgen. The secondary form may arise from a disorder outside the adrenal glands such as a pituitary tumour. Graves' disease is an immune system disorder that results in the overproduction of thyroid hormones (hyperthyroidism). Although several disorders may result in hyperthyroidism, Graves' disease is a common cause. Hypothyroidism occurs when the thyroid gland is underactive, producing insufficient amounts of thyroid hormone. Goitre is an enlargement of the thyroid gland, which can be caused by a lack of iodine in the diet or can arise sporadically because of exposure to certain foods or drugs. Goitre can be classified as toxic or non-toxic.

13 **Cushing's syndrome is characterized by an excess of which type of hormone?**

a) antidiuretic hormone

b) glucagon

c) *glucocorticoid*

d) aldosterone

Cushing's syndrome is caused when the adrenal glands secrete excess amounts of the glucocorticoid hormones and sometimes excess androgens as well. In most patients, Cushing's syndrome is the result of an oversecretion of corticotropin, which causes excessive cell proliferation in the adrenal cortex.

14 **Which of the following is *not* a chronic complication of pheochromocytoma?**
a) persistent hypertension   b) glucose intolerance
c) hypermetabolism   ***d) anhidrosis***

Pheochromocytomas are tumours derived from the chromaffin cells of the adrenal medulla resulting in adrenomedullary hyperfunction. Symptoms of the condition are related to the effects of chronic catecholamine secretion and include persistent hypertension and associated diaphoresis, tachycardia, palpitations and severe headaches. Glucose intolerance frequently results from catecholamine-induced inhibition of pancreatic insulin. Hypermetabolism is related to chronic activation of sympathetic receptors in adipocytes and hepatocytes, although other tissues may be involved.

15 **Which of the following is a symptom of hypothyroidism?**
a) diarrhoea   ***b) constipation***
c) sensitivity to heat   d) unexplained weight loss

Constipation is a symptom of hypothyroidism due to the suppression of metabolic activity which slows motility in the gastrointestinal (GI) tract. Diarrhoea occurs when motility in the GI tract is too fast. Other symptoms of hypothyroidism include sensitivity to cold, numbness or tingling, muscle cramps, joint stiffness, tremors/poor coordination, dry skin, anaemia, fertility problems, high cholesterol weight gain due to fatigue and reduced activity.

FILL IN THE BLANKS

16 ***Ketoacidosis* is recognized as a serious acute complication of diabetes mellitus.**
Ketoacidosis is a serious complication of diabetes mellitus and a common cause of medical emergency in diabetic patients. The condition presents when there is an absolute or relative deficiency

in insulin. In a state of relative insulin insufficiency, there is an increase in the insulin counterregulatory hormones which antagonize insulin by increasing insulin production and reducing use of glucose. Profound insulin deficiency results in decreased glucose uptake, increased fat metabolism and accelerated gluconeogenesis and ketogenesis, resulting in the increased production of acidic ketone bodies and insufficient buffering of the circulation. This results most commonly in the characteristic hyperventilation that attempts to compensate for the acidosis (Kussmaul respirations), CNS depression, ketonuria, anorexia, nausea, thirst and polyuria.

17 **A patient with _Addison's_ disease would exhibit symptoms including weight loss, dehydration and a craving for salty food.**
Other symptoms of this disease include fatigue, GI disturbances, muscle weakness, faintness, anxiety and (in pre-menopausal females) amenorrhoea. Patients can be treated with hydrocortisone and aldosterone and may expect to live a normal lifespan.

18 **A complication of _Cushing's_ disease is associated hypertension which can lead to ischaemic heart disease.**
This is quite common in Cushing's disease and can ultimately lead to heart failure. Other complications include osteoporosis caused by increased calcium resorption from bones, peptic ulcers due to increased gastric secretions, and impaired glucose tolerance caused by insulin resistance.

19 **_Glucagon_ stimulates hepatic glucose production and release of glucose into the circulation during periods of hypoglycaemia.**
Glucagon is a peptide hormone, produced by alpha cells of the pancreas. It raises the concentration of glucose and fatty acids in the circulation and is the main catabolic hormone of the body. The pancreas releases glucagon when the amount of glucose in the bloodstream is abnormally low. Glucagon causes the liver to initiate glycogenolysis: converting stored glycogen into glucose, which is released into the circulation. High blood glucose levels, on the other hand, stimulate the release of insulin. Insulin allows glucose to be taken up and used by insulin-dependent tissues. Thus, glucagon and insulin are part of a feedback system that keeps blood glucose levels stable. Glucagon increases energy expenditure and is elevated under conditions of stress. It is also used as a medication to treat several health conditions, including low blood sugar, beta

blocker overdose, calcium channel blocker toxicity and anaphylaxis refractory to epinephrine.

20 | **Blindness, end-stage renal failure and neuropathy are leading complications of diabetic _microvascular_ disease.**

Microvascular complications of diabetes are those long-term complications that affect the small blood vessels. These typically include retinopathy, nephropathy and neuropathy. *Retinopathy* is divided into two main categories: non-proliferative and proliferative. Non-proliferative retinopathy relates to the development of microaneurysms, venous loops, retinal haemorrhages, hard exudates and soft exudates. Proliferative retinopathy identifies the presence of new blood vessels, with or without vitreous haemorrhage and can be considered a progression of non-proliferative retinopathy. Diabetic *nephropathy* is defined as persistent proteinuria. It can progress to overt nephropathy characterized by a progressive decline in renal function resulting in end-stage renal disease. *Neuropathy* is a heterogeneous condition associated with nerve pathology. The condition is classified according to the nerves affected and includes focal, diffuse, sensory, motor and autonomic neuropathy.

In contrast, the macrovascular complications of diabetes are primarily diseases of the coronary arteries, peripheral arteries and cerebral vasculature. Early macrovascular disease is associated with atherosclerotic plaque in the vasculature supplying blood to the heart, brain, limbs and other organs. Late stages of macrovascular disease involve complete obstruction of these vessels, which can increase the risks of myocardial infarction (MI), stroke, claudication and gangrene. Cardiovascular disease (CVD) is the major cause of morbidity and mortality in patients with diabetes.

PUZZLE GRID

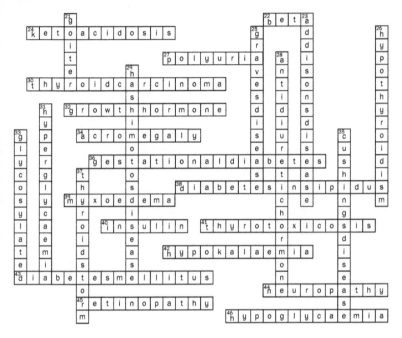

5 The cardiovascular system

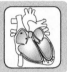

INTRODUCTION

The heart and blood provide all the organs and tissues with nutrients and oxygen and remove waste. Diseases and disorders of the cardiovascular system may affect the heart, the blood and/or blood vessels and may be primary disorders of the system – such as myocardial infarction (MI) or cerebrovascular accident (CVA) – or secondary disorders caused by a condition arising in another organ system (for example, septicaemia arising as a complication of cellulitis).

Many of the signs and symptoms of cardiovascular system disorders are initially general and vague. Often when specific symptoms arise and the patient presents for treatment, the damage to the heart and vessels of the circulatory system is irreversible. Acute cardiovascular disorders (MI or CVA) are considered medical emergencies because they can be life-threatening if not accurately diagnosed and treated rapidly.

Disorders of the cardiovascular system affect many people during their lifetime, but many are preventable through lifestyle adjustments, so patient education has an important role in helping reduce the incidence of such conditions and maintaining quality of life for the patients affected. Public health campaigns now focus on raising awareness of disorders of this system, to help people reduce their risk of developing cardiovascular disease. In many instances, awareness and simple lifestyle adjustments may reduce risks and significantly improve life expectancy.

Nurses should appreciate that chronic or acute disruption or damage to the organs or vessels of the cardiovascular system can have serious and life-threatening consequences.

Useful resources

Nurses! Test Yourself in Anatomy and Physiology (2nd edition)
Chapter 5

Ross and Wilson's Anatomy and Physiology in Health and Illness (14th edition)
Chapters 4 and 5

TRUE OR FALSE?

Are the following statements true or false?

1   All veins have corresponding arteries that run alongside each other.

2   If the heart valves become damaged, abnormal murmurs can be heard.

3   Cardiovascular disease describes disorders of the heart and its surrounding blood vessels.

4   The normal range for blood pH is 7.35–7.45.

5   Hypertension is a decrease in blood pressure.

6   Hypertension is a symptom of shock.

7   An aneurysm is an abnormal narrowing of an arterial wall.

8   Aneurysms are often asymptomatic.

9   Heart failure occurs as a result of impaired atrial function due to abnormality of the myocardial muscle.

| 10 | When the atria distend in heart failure, there is a reflexive decrease in heart rate. |

| 11 | Myocardial infarction (heart attack) is an acute coronary syndrome. |

| 12 | Stable angina is classified as an acute coronary syndrome. |

MULTIPLE CHOICE

Identify one correct answer for each of the following:

13 Anaemia is caused by a deficiency of which essential element?

a) iron

b) oxygen

c) nitrogen

d) carbon

14 The immediate treatment for shock is:

a) give the patient a drink to calm him/her down

b) administer oxygen

c) identify the cause of the shock before administering treatment

d) lie the patient down with feet above the head

15 Which of the following is *not* a form of circulatory shock?

a) septic shock

b) cardiogenic shock

c) psychological shock

d) obstructive shock

16 Coronary artery disease occurs when:

a) the body's glucose supply exceeds demand

b) the body's water demand exceeds supply

c) the body's oxygen demand exceeds supply

d) the body's oxygen supply exceeds demand

17 The main symptom of coronary artery disease is:

a) angina

b) breathlessness

c) cerebrovascular accident

d) headache

18 Which of the following is *not* a predisposing risk factor for myocardial infarction?

a) diabetes mellitus

b) elevated serum lipid levels

c) hypertension

d) cerebrovascular accident

19 Susceptibility to complications from myocardial infarction increases with:

a) age

b) body weight

c) serum lipid levels

d) hypertension

20 How long does it take for cardiac troponins T and I to become elevated after a myocardial infarction?

a) within 30 seconds

b) within 10 minutes

c) within 4–6 hours

d) within 1–2 weeks

21 Which of these tests would identify the cause and severity of heart failure?

a) cardiac enzymes

b) echocardiogram

c) electrocardiogram

d) X-ray

22 Heart failure can usually be treated quickly with which type of drug?

a) anticoagulants

b) antiplatelet medications

c) beta-adrenoceptor blockers

d) diuretics

23 Which of these drug classes are used to prevent aneurysm rupture?

a) ACE-inhibitors

b) aspirin

c) beta-adrenoceptor blockers

d) nonsteroidal anti-inflammatory drugs

FILL IN THE BLANKS

Fill in the blanks in each statement using the options in this box.
Not all of them are required, so choose carefully!

myeloid	pacemaker	irreversible
reduced	electrocardiogram	preserved
MRI	CVA	lymphoid
atherosclerosis	hypertension	cardiac marker
pulmonary embolism	lymphocytic	lymphocytic

24 Systolic heart failure is also classified as heart failure with _____ ejection fraction.

25 Diastolic heart failure can be classified as heart failure with _____ ejection fraction.

26 _____ does not produce any signs or symptoms until vascular damage has occurred in the heart, brain or kidneys.

27 The formation of atheroma on the inner walls of coronary arteries is called _____.

28 An artificial _____ may be fitted to stabilize arrhythmias following a myocardial infarction.

29 An _____ is the main tool used to diagnose angina or myocardial infarction.

30 A _____ _____ may develop as a complication of deep vein thrombosis.

31 _____ _____ enzymes are proteins used to diagnose myocardial infarction.

32 Leukaemia can be classified as acute or chronic and _____ or _____.

33 Chronic _____ leukaemia is the slowest and most benign form of leukaemia.

34 The _____ phase of shock cannot be corrected, even with medical intervention.

PUZZLE GRID

Use the word bank (below) and clues (overleaf) to solve the puzzle.

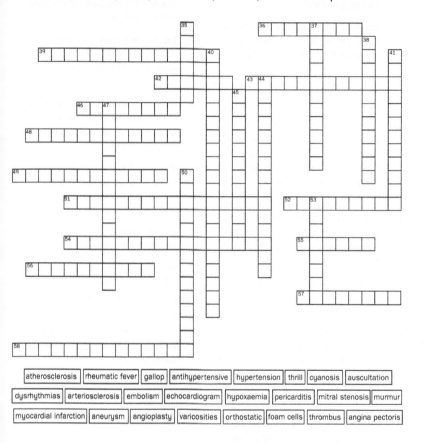

atherosclerosis | rheumatic fever | gallop | antihypertensive | hypertension | thrill | cyanosis | auscultation

dysrhythmias | arteriosclerosis | embolism | echocardiogram | hypoxaemia | pericarditis | mitral stenosis | murmur

myocardial infarction | aneurysm | angioplasty | varicosities | orthostatic | foam cells | thrombus | angina pectoris

Clues across

36 Bluish-purple discoloration of the skin or mucous membranes caused by deoxygenated or reduced haemoglobin in the blood (8)

39 Type of ultrasound scan used to look at the heart and nearby blood vessels (14)

Clues down

35 Palpable vibration associated with a cardiac murmur and certain other cardiac or respiratory conditions (6)

37 Rapid drop in blood pressure associated with a sudden change in position; postural hypotension (11)

95

Clues across (continued)

42 Abnormal rhythm of the heart that presents with three or four sounds on auscultation (6)

43 Twisted, swollen and raised veins at the skin's surface that may have a bluish-purple or red colour (12)

46 Blood clot formed *in situ* within the vascular system that restricts blood flow (8)

48 Long-term medical condition in which arterial blood pressure is consistently elevated, increasing the risk of stroke, cardiac failure, chronic kidney disease and dementia (12)

49 Procedure performed for the purpose of examining the internal sounds of the body, usually using a stethoscope (12)

51 Class of drug used to reduce complications of long-term elevated blood pressure (16)

52 Type of macrophage that localize to fatty deposits on blood vessel walls, where they ingest low-density lipoproteins and become laden with lipids (4, 5)

54 Thickening, hardening and loss of elasticity of the walls of arteries; primary cause of coronary artery disease (16)

Clues down (continued)

38 Medical procedure that opens a blocked or narrowed artery around the heart; percutaneous coronary intervention (11)

40 Medical emergency in which the supply of blood to the heart is suddenly reduced or blocked; heart attack (10, 10)

41 Disturbances in the rate of cardiac muscle contractions that may occur through ventricular tachycardia or atrial fibrillation (12)

44 Build-up of fats, cholesterol and other substances in and on the arterial walls leading to hardening and narrowing of the vessel (15)

45 Inflammation of the serous membranes of the heart (12)

47 Complication of bacterial throat infections associated with painful joints and heart problems (9, 5)

50 Form of valvular heart disease characterized by an accumulation of blood in the heart and fluid in the lungs (6, 8)

53 Bulge in an artery caused by a weakness in the blood vessel wall (8)

Clues across (continued)

55 Sounds made by turbulent blood in or near the heart that can be heard on auscultation (6)

56 Decrease in the partial pressure of oxygen in the blood that may occur through V/Q mismatch, right-to-left shunt, diffusion impairment, hypoventilation or low inspired PO_2 (10)

57 Blocked artery caused by a foreign body, such as a blood clot or an air bubble (8)

58 Type of chest pain caused by reduced blood flow to the heart; symptom of coronary artery disease (6, 8)

ANSWERS

TRUE OR FALSE?

1 | **All veins have corresponding arteries that run alongside each other.**

Deep veins have corresponding arteries that are usually located alongside each other; more superficial veins do not have corresponding arteries. At any given time, the majority of blood in the body is being transported through deep veins. Although most veins take blood back to the heart, there is an exception – the hepatic portal vein. Damage to this vein can be dangerous. Blood clotting in the hepatic portal vein can cause portal hypertension, which results in a decrease of blood flow to the liver.

2 | **If the heart valves become damaged, abnormal murmurs can be heard.**

The heart valves can be damaged through injury or disease (such as endocarditis or rheumatic fever), although damage is more commonly due to congenital abnormalities. Additional murmurs can be heard as the blood flows forwards through narrowed valves or leaks backwards through incompetent valves. Symptoms associated with aortic valve damage may not present until the damage is quite advanced. They include angina (because the heart is working harder to pump blood away) and dyspnoea, dizziness and fainting (all associated with the obstruction of blood flow from the heart). Abnormal murmurs can usually be detected with a stethoscope and require referral for further investigation.

3 | **Cardiovascular disease describes disorders of the heart and its surrounding blood vessels.**

Cardiovascular diseases are diseases of the heart or blood vessels (vasculature). However, the term 'cardiovascular disease' is often used to describe diseases of the heart or blood vessels that are caused by atheroma (also known as atherosclerosis or hardening of the arteries). Patches of atheroma are small fatty lumps (or plaques) that develop on the inner, endothelial lining of arteries.

Cardiovascular diseases that can be caused by atheroma include angina, MI, CVA and peripheral vascular disease.

4 | **The normal range for blood pH is 7.35–7.45.**
The normal pH range of circulating blood is maintained by buffer systems, the lungs and the kidneys. When these systems are functioning normally together, they neutralize and eliminate acids as quickly as they are formed.

5 | **Hypertension is a decrease in blood pressure.**
Hypertension is an intermittent or sustained elevation of resting systolic and/or diastolic blood pressure (BP). It is caused by increases in cardiac output and/or peripheral resistance, making the heart work more. A resting systolic BP of greater than 140 mmHg is said to be high, while a resting diastolic BP of greater than 90 mmHg is considered high. Therefore, a BP of 140/90 mmHg is said to be elevated. A BP of 120/100 mmHg is indicative of an elevated diastolic BP (since the systolic value is within the normal range), whereas a BP of 160/60 mmHg is indicative of a high systolic pressure (since the diastolic value is within the normal range). Patients who have a sustained high BP are usually prescribed medication to help lower it. Hypertension is a risk factor for cardiovascular disease and kidney damage because sustained elevated blood pressure puts strain on the arteries, the heart and the delicate kidney vessels.

6 | **Hypertension is a symptom of shock.**
Shock is an acute condition caused when the circulatory system fails, depriving the tissues of oxygen and nutrients and indicated by hypotension (low blood pressure). This is circulatory (or physiological) shock and should not be confused with emotional shock. Circulatory shock can be severe and potentially life-threatening. It can be caused by: (1) a fall in cardiac output after a haemorrhage or other fluid loss; (2) damage to the heart after a MI; (3) external pressure on the heart; or (4) extensive peripheral vasodilation such as in an anaphylactic hypersensitivity reaction. Other symptoms of shock include pale or clammy skin, confusion/disorientation, rapid shallow breathing, rapid weak pulse, nausea or vomiting, and thirst. Respiratory acidosis may develop as a complication due to the drop in blood pH (see Chapter 6, Answer 8).

7 **An aneurysm is an abnormal narrowing of an arterial wall.** ✗

An aneurysm is abnormal dilation (stretching or widening) of an arterial wall. Aneurysms can occur in the brain (cerebral or intracranial aneurysm) or aorta (known as abdominal aortic aneurysm). In an abdominal aortic aneurysm, this dilation occurs in the aorta between the renal arteries and the iliac branches. Aneurysms are more common in males than females. They usually develop due to a muscular weakness in the artery wall that allows the vessel to stretch outward. Blood pressure (especially high BP) can weaken the vessel wall and increase the size of the aneurysm. Narrowing of arterial walls is caused by accumulation of atherosclerotic plaques (atheroma) on the inner layer (intima) of the walls of the coronary arteries. When a blood clot attaches to atheroma, blood supply to cardiac tissue can be reduced and this may result in angina or an MI (see Figures 5.1 and 5.2).

Figure 5.1 Myocardial infarction

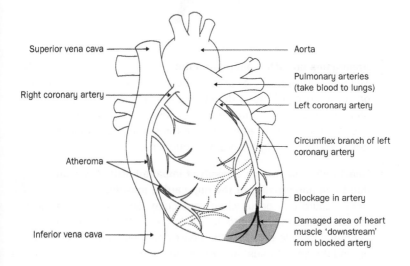

Superior vena cava

Aorta

Pulmonary arteries (take blood to lungs)

Right coronary artery

Left coronary artery

Circumflex branch of left coronary artery

Atheroma

Blockage in artery

Damaged area of heart muscle 'downstream' from blocked artery

Inferior vena cava

Figure 5.2 Section of an occluded coronary artery causing an MI

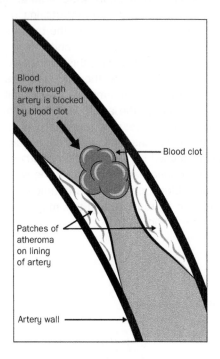

8 | **Aneurysms are often asymptomatic.**
Many aneurysms do not produce symptoms and are only detected on an X-ray or CT scan during routine physical examination or if there is a family history. In many cases, the exact cause of an aneurysm is unclear, although risk factors include smoking, hypertension and a family history of aneurysms.

9 | **Heart failure occurs as a result of impaired atrial function due to an abnormality of the myocardial muscle.**
Heart failure can occur when ventricular function (usually the left ventricle) is impaired due to cardiac muscle abnormalities. This abnormal muscle prevents the heart from pumping sufficient blood around the body to sustain oxygen and nutrient requirements of the tissues. The main symptom of heart failure is extreme tiredness due to the lack of oxygen getting to muscles and tissues. Other symptoms depend on the side of the heart affected.

Left-sided heart failure is more common and will cause dyspnoea (breathlessness) due to the accumulation of fluid in the blood vessels of the lungs (pulmonary congestion). Right-sided heart failure can cause oedema in the ankles, legs and abdomen due to accumulation of excess fluid in the veins that return blood to the heart; this increases blood pressure in the veins, which pushes fluid out of the veins and into the surrounding tissues, causing peripheral swelling, particularly in the lower extremities. Fluid can also accumulate in the liver and stomach. Symptoms associated with failure on either side (or both sides) of the heart include dizziness, loss of appetite, nausea and constipation.

10 **When the atria distend in heart failure, there is a reflexive decrease in heart rate.**

When the atria distend, there is a reflexive increase in the heart rate to pump the extra blood returning to the heart in venous return. Atrial distension can occur in heart failure or due to over-transfusion. When there is a sudden reduction in the pressure in the atria, the heartbeat slows. This is called the Bainbridge reflex and is the cause of the significant bradycardia sometimes seen during spinal anaesthesia. It is best treated by elevating the legs to increase the venous return.

11 **Myocardial infarction (heart attack) is an acute coronary syndrome.**

Acute coronary syndrome (ACS) is a term used to describe a range of thrombotic coronary artery diseases that cause acute ischaemia of the myocardial muscle tissue, namely unstable angina, ST-elevation MI (STEMI) and non-ST-elevation MI (non-STEMI). All of these conditions are described as ACS because they reduce or impede blood flow through one of the coronary arteries causing ischaemia, injury and necrosis (infarction) to the tissue around the heart (see Figure 5.1). STEMI is the most serious ACS event because of the prolonged interruption of blood supply to the heart tissue, usually because the artery is completely occluded (blocked) (see Figure 5.2). A non-STEMI is less severe because the artery is only partly blocked, meaning blood supply is reduced but not completely impeded, and therefore only part of the heart muscle being supplied by the affected artery is threatened. The different types of MI are diagnosed based on ECG observations (see Figure 5.3). Signs and symptoms of ACS are similar and are usually diagnosed from a detailed patient (and family) history, physical examination, electrocardiogram (ECG) and serum cardiac marker (enzyme) studies. ACS is a medical emergency and requires immediate hospital admission.

Figure 5.3 ECG patterns in MI

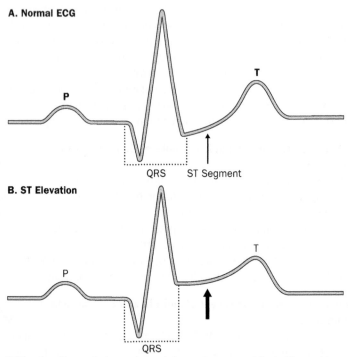

A. Normal ECG

P

T

QRS   ST Segment

B. ST Elevation

P

T

QRS

ST Elevation: Observed when acute heart damage has occurred due to MI – would indicate a STEMI.

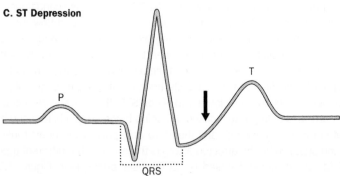

C. ST Depression

P

T

QRS

ST Depression: indicates ischaemia has occurred but is not a sign of infarction. Patient may experience pain. T wave may also be flattened or inverted. Treatment with digoxin can produce ST depression and inverted T wave.

This pattern is also caused by biochemical conditions such as hypokalaemia, Hypocalcaemia or hypomagnesaemia and may be observed in cases of hypothermia.

12 | **Stable angina is classified as an acute coronary syndrome.** ✗

Stable angina is not a symptom of acute coronary syndrome because it is not life-threatening. However, it is an important warning sign of an increased risk of more serious conditions, such as MI or CVA. Unstable angina, in contrast, is a symptom of acute coronary syndrome because symptoms develop rapidly, can persist even at rest, and can last up to 30 minutes. It is much more likely to develop into an MI than stable angina. It can sometimes be relieved by nitrates (such as glyceryl trinitrate, or GTN), which relax and dilate the blood vessels, increasing the blood supply to the heart. However, sometimes angina can be resistant to this treatment. Upon admission to hospital, patients are usually administered anticoagulant medication (such as heparin) to prevent MI. Other drugs can be used to control and reduce the risk of acute coronary disease, including beta-adrenoceptor blockers (beta-blockers) or angiotensin-converting enzyme (ACE) inhibitors as well as statins to control serum cholesterol levels.

MULTIPLE CHOICE
Correct answers identified in ***bold italics***

13 | **Anaemia is caused by a deficiency of which essential element?**

a) iron   b) oxygen   c) nitrogen   d) carbon

If there is a lack of iron in the diet, a patient can develop anaemia, which means the production of haemoglobin is reduced, which affects the ability of the red blood cells to carry and distribute oxygen around the body. In the UK, normal haemoglobin levels are in the range of 130–170 g/L in males and 120–150 g/L in females. Values in children vary with age. Other causes of anaemia include pregnancy, excess blood loss (perhaps due to bleeding ulcer or injury) or conditions that result in poor iron absorption from food. Symptoms usually include fatigue, poor concentration, tachycardia and paleness (especially of the conjunctivae and nail beds). Treatment usually involves an oral iron supplement (sometimes in combination with ascorbic acid – vitamin C – which enhances iron absorption) and dietary advice to increase iron consumption.

14 **The immediate treatment for shock is:**

a) give the patient a drink to calm him/her down

b) administer oxygen

c) identify the cause of the shock before administering treatment

d) lie the patient down with feet above the head

Ideally the feet should be elevated above the head, which will help raise the blood pressure and preserve blood flow to the brain. If the brain is starved of oxygen, the tissue will begin to die and damage will be irreversible. Treatment should also aim to stop any bleeding by applying direct pressure over the wound or a tourniquet on extreme limb injuries. A patient suffering from suspected shock should never be given anything to eat or drink because of the risk of vomiting. If the patient is experiencing anaphylactic shock and is conscious but having trouble breathing, it is best to sit them upright.

15 **Which of the following is *not* a form of circulatory shock?**

a) septic shock

b) cardiogenic shock

c) psychological shock

d) obstructive shock

Psychological (emotional) shock should not be confused with circulatory (or physiological) shock. Psychological shock can occur after a physically or emotionally traumatic experience and affects the state of mind. It can produce symptoms such as palpitations and faintness, but it does not usually lead to serious physical collapse. Septic shock, cardiogenic shock and obstructive shock are forms of circulatory shock that are not caused by low blood volume but are still life-threatening. Septic shock is caused by bacteria releasing massive amounts of toxins during a systemic infection, causing peripheral vasodilation and a dangerous drop in blood pressure. Symptoms are similar to other circulatory shocks, but patients may exhibit a fever due to the infection. Cardiogenic shock occurs when the heart is unable to maintain a normal cardiac output – often caused by a failure in the left ventricle after MI. Thrombolytic (clot-busting) drugs can restore coronary circulation and relieve symptoms. Other causes of cardiogenic shock include arrhythmias, valve disorders and advanced coronary heart disease. Obstructive shock occurs upon ventricular output being reduced when fluid or tissue restricts the beating of the heart. It is often caused by fluid build-up in the pericardial cavity (cardiac tamponade).

16 **Coronary artery disease occurs when:**
a) the body's glucose supply exceeds demand
b) the body's water demand exceeds supply
c) ***the body's oxygen demand exceeds supply***
d) the body's oxygen supply exceeds demand

Coronary artery disease (CAD) reduces the supply of oxygen and nutrients to myocardial tissues due to poor coronary blood flow. The most common cause of CAD is atherosclerosis, when fatty, fibrous plaques (atheroma) accumulate. This narrows the inner lining of the walls of arteries supplying the heart, thus reducing the volume of blood that can flow through the vessels. Many of the risk factors associated with CAD are modifiable, so patients can help to reduce their risks of developing CAD, or the associated MI, by making minor lifestyle adjustments, such as eating a diet low in saturated fat and taking regular moderate exercise.

17 **The main symptom of coronary artery disease is:**
a) ***angina***   b) breathlessness
c) cerebrovascular accident   d) headache

Angina is a classic sign of CAD. Patients may report a crushing, squeezing or burning pain in the left side of the chest that radiates down the left arm and sometimes upwards into the neck and jaw – the same type of pain experienced in MI. The pain is often accompanied by nausea, vomiting, fainting or sweating, although not all patients, especially females, report the classic pain symptoms of angina or MI. Symptoms usually occur after physical exertion or high emotions but can develop during rest or even sleep.

18 **Which of the following is *not* a predisposing risk factor for myocardial infarction?**
a) diabetes mellitus   b) elevated serum lipid levels
c) hypertension   d) ***cerebrovascular accident***

A history of CVA is not associated with increased risk of MI. MI is caused by an occlusion (blockage) of a coronary artery; the occlusion can be due to one of several factors, such as atherosclerosis, thrombosis or platelet aggregation (clumping). Many of the predisposing factors for MI or ACS are lifestyle-related and include a sedentary lifestyle, high salt diet, obesity, smoking, stress and the use of recreational drugs. Non-lifestyle factors include increasing age and a family history of coronary artery disease.

19 **Susceptibility to complications from myocardial infarction increases with:**

a)   age   b)   body weight
c)   serum lipid levels   d)   hypertension

Risk of complications and death associated with MI increases with a person's age. Complications include arrhythmias, cardiogenic shock or heart failure, causing pulmonary oedema, or rupture of chamber walls or valves.

20 **How long does it take for cardiac troponins T and I to become elevated after a myocardial infarction?**

a)   within 30 seconds   b)   within 10 minutes
c)   within 4–6 hours   d)   within 1–2 weeks

The cardiac troponins (cTn) T and I are proteins that are released within 4–6 hours of a MI and peak between 24 and 48 hours. They remain elevated above baseline levels for up to 2 weeks after the attack and are almost completely specific to myocardial tissue. Therefore, they are the preferred markers for assessing myocardial damage over other cardiac enzymes such as creatine kinase (CK), aspartate aminotransferase (AST) or lactate dehydrogenase (LAD), which all have much lower specificity for cardiac muscle than troponins T and I. Troponin is a contractile protein not normally found in serum. It is only released when myocardial necrosis occurs. Cardiac troponins T and I are highly sensitive and specific to myocardial tissue damage. Troponins T and I are of equal clinical value; when elevated troponins are detected along with chest pain, it is considered a strong predictor of MI in the near future. The risk of death from ACS is directly related to troponin levels; patients with no detectable troponins have a positive short-term prognosis.

21 **Which of these tests would identify the cause and severity of heart failure?**

a)   cardiac enzymes   *b)   echocardiogram*
c)   electrocardiogram   d)   X-ray

An echocardiogram is an ultrasound scan that evaluates the pumping action of the heart. It will help identify the underlying cause, type and severity of heart failure. A chest X-ray will determine if the heart is enlarged and if there is fluid in the lungs, while an ECG records the electrical activity and rhythms of the heart. A number of cardiac enzymes are released by the myocardial cells following damage due to MI.

22 **Heart failure can usually be treated quickly with which type of drug?**

a) anticoagulants　　　　　　　b) antiplatelet medications
c) beta-adrenoceptor blockers　　***d) diuretics***

The immediate treatment of heart failure usually consists of a combination of diuretics and vasodilators. Diuretics such as furosemide are administered to reduce blood volume and the resulting congestion in the circulatory system. Vasodilators (namely ACE-inhibitors) allow the arteries to relax and dilate and increase cardiac output, making it easier for the heart to pump blood around the body. Anticoagulants, such as warfarin, and antiplatelet treatment, such as aspirin, thin the blood and therefore help prevent stroke. These are recommended for the management of chronic heart failure but should not be used in combination because their combined effects may cause haemorrhage. Beta-adrenoceptor blockers are not commonly used to treat heart failure in an emergency but can be used in long-term management of chronic heart failure.

23 **Which of these drug classes are used to prevent aneurysm rupture?**

a) ACE-inhibitors
b) aspirin
c) beta-adrenoceptor blockers
d) nonsteroidal anti-inflammatory drugs

Beta-adrenoceptor blockers (beta-blockers) are usually prescribed to decrease the extension of an aneurysm and prevent rupture, but surgery may be required if the aneurysm is quite large or at risk of rupture. An alternative to surgical resection (removal) of the aneurysm is a stent graft, where the damaged section of the blood vessel is replaced with a piece of supportive tubing. Symptoms of a ruptured aneurysm include sweating, weakness and tachycardia. A ruptured aortic aneurysm will also be accompanied by severe abdominal pain. If left untreated, a ruptured aneurysm will result in death, although before shock sets in, patients may remain quite stable for a number of hours before death. A ruptured aortic aneurysm will be fatal in 65–85% of patients.

FILL IN THE BLANKS

24 **Systolic heart failure is also classified as heart failure with _reduced_ ejection fraction.**
The heart's ejection fraction refers to the amount (percentage) of blood pumped out (or ejected) from the left ventricle with each contraction. Systolic heart failure is considered to be a 'pumping problem' that occurs when the left ventricle cannot contract vigorously enough to maintain adequate circulation in the systemic circulation. The cardiac muscle is weakened and no longer capable of pumping the blood around the body when it contracts, therefore, there is a decrease in the supply of oxygen to the organs, tissues and cells of the body. This is known as reduced ejection fraction.

25 **Diastolic heart failure can be classified as heart failure with _preserved_ ejection fraction.**
In heart failure with preserved ejection fraction, the cardiac muscle is still strong and pumping blood around the body at an adequate force. However, after pumping the blood from the ventricle, the left ventricle cannot relax and widen fully to allow it to fill again, so insufficient blood is pumped out of the heart, especially during strenuous exercise. This 'filling problem' is characteristic of diastolic heart failure because the heart muscle should be relaxing and widening during the diastolic phase.

26 **_Hypertension_ does not produce any signs or symptoms until vascular damage has occurred in the heart, brain or kidneys.**
Hypertension is asymptomatic (has no symptoms) when it first begins but if left untreated, sustained hypertension damages the lining of blood vessels and can produce major complications that can be fatal. Symptoms that may develop include transient ischaemic attack (TIA) or stroke, while blindness can develop due to damage to the blood vessels of the retina. Hypertension can cause an MI while prolonged protein in urine (proteinuria) and oedema can result in renal failure.

27 **The formation of atheroma on the inner walls of coronary arteries is called _atherosclerosis_.**
Atherosclerosis is a form of arteriosclerosis characterized by the deposition of atheroma containing cholesterol and lipids on the

innermost membrane (*tunica intima*) of the walls of large and medium-sized arteries. Individuals with atherosclerosis have a higher risk of coronary artery disease and stroke. Smoking, hypertension, diabetes mellitus, as well as elevated levels of saturated fat in the blood contribute to the development of atherosclerosis. Arteriosclerosis describes the thickening, hardening and loss of elasticity of the arterial walls that results in impaired blood circulation; it is associated with increasing age as well as hypertension, diabetes mellitus and poor diet.

28 **An artificial _pacemaker_ may be fitted to stabilize arrhythmias following a myocardial infarction.**

Arrhythmias are the most common problem immediately after MI and stabilizing these is one of the three goals of MI treatment. The others are to relieve chest pain and reduce the workload of the heart. A pacemaker may be fitted temporarily to stabilize heart beat and treat life-threatening bradycardia. To relieve chest pain, a patient would usually be treated with IV morphine and beta-blockers to reduce the workload of the heart. In addition, patients may be prescribed statins if their serum cholesterol levels are elevated.

29 **An _electrocardiogram_ is the main tool used to diagnose angina or myocardial infarction.**

An ECG can be used to diagnose angina and will show ischaemia in the form of an inverted T-wave, ST-segment depression and possibly arrhythmias (Figure 5.3).

30 **A _pulmonary embolism_ may develop as a complication of deep vein thrombosis.**

Deep vein thrombosis (DVT) is a blood clot in one of the deep veins in the body, usually a deep leg vein that runs through the muscles of the calf and thigh. It can cause pain and swelling in the leg. Complications such as pulmonary embolism may arise when a piece of blood clot breaks off, travels in the bloodstream and blocks one of the blood vessels in the lungs. DVT and pulmonary embolism together are known as venous thromboembolism (VTE). Anyone can develop DVT, although there are some particular risk factors, such as a family history of thrombosis, pregnancy, medical conditions (cancer or heart failure), inactivity (for example, after an operation) and obesity. Sometimes DVT may be asymptomatic, although symptoms include pain, swelling and a heavy ache in the leg, a warm feeling around the affected area and redness on the skin around the area. Symptoms of a pulmonary embolism are more serious and include breathlessness, which may come on gradually or suddenly, chest pain, which may be worse when inhaling, or sudden collapse. If symptoms of DVT or pulmonary embolism develop, urgent medical attention should be sought as these conditions may be life-threatening. DVT is usually treated with anticoagulants such as warfarin or heparin. Heparin may be used in emergencies to thin the blood and is suitable for use during pregnancy (whereas warfarin is not). Patients will also be advised to elevate their leg and wear compression stockings to relieve pressure on the leg veins and prevent fluid accumulation in the calf.

| 31 | ***Cardiac marker* enzymes are proteins used to diagnose myocardial infarction.** |

Diagnosis of MI requires two of three components, namely history, ECG and cardiac marker enzymes. When damage to the heart occurs, levels of cardiac markers rise over time, which is why blood tests are taken over a 24-hour period. The specific enzymes that are measured to diagnose MI are creatinine kinase (CK) and cardiac troponins. Troponins T and I are specific to myocardial injury, although these enzyme levels are not elevated immediately following MI. If patients present with chest pain, they are generally treated on the assumption that MI has occurred and then evaluated over time for a more precise diagnosis.

| 32 | **Leukaemia can be classified as acute or chronic and *lymphoid* or *myeloid.*** |

Leukaemia describes a group of malignant disorders of the white blood cells (WBCs). In acute leukaemias, immature WBCs accumulate in the body and disrupt the function of organs and tissues. In chronic leukaemias, cells are slightly abnormal and therefore do not function properly. Lymphoid refers to lymphocytes (type of white blood cell) that arise from lymphoid stem cells while the remaining WBCs arise from myeloid stem cells. Risks associated with acute leukaemias are increased by smoking, exposure to radiation and treatment for a previous cancer diagnosis. Symptoms for all leukaemias are vague and include fatigue, weight loss, frequent infections and anaemia. If untreated, acute leukaemias progress rapidly and aggressively. They can be fatal and prognosis varies with treatment and type of disease. Acute lymphocytic leukaemia (ALL) accounts for about 80% of childhood leukaemias, while acute myeloid leukaemia (AML) is one of the most common leukaemias in adults.

33 **Chronic _lymphocytic_ leukaemia is the slowest and most benign form of leukaemia.**

Chronic lymphocytic leukaemia (CLL) is a progressive disease that causes a proliferation and accumulation of malfunctioning, immune-deficient lymphocytes. Risk increases with age and hereditary factors are thought to be involved in CLL, which is more common in males. Chronic myeloid leukaemia (CML) is caused by excessive development of granulocytes in the bone marrow, which circulate in the blood and infiltrate the liver and spleen. CML risk increases with age and exposure to radiation and carcinogenic chemicals (such as benzene). Some signs and symptoms for both types of chronic leukaemia are similar to acute leukaemias and include fatigue, weight loss and frequent infections. For chronic leukaemias, there may also be swelling of lymph glands, liver and enlargement of the spleen (splenomegaly). Tests for CLL usually include a lymph node biopsy, which distinguishes benign and malignant tumours, while routine blood tests will usually identify an increasing lympho-cyte count along with low haemoglobin levels. Tests for CML would include a bone marrow biopsy to check for bone marrow infiltration along with WBC count. CT scans would identify affected organs and tissues.

34 **The _irreversible_ phase of shock cannot be corrected, even with medical intervention.**

In the absence of treatment, circulatory shock will progress into irreversible (or refractory) shock when the heart, liver, kidneys and central nervous system rapidly begin to deteriorate and eventu-ally fail. This cannot be reversed, even with medical intervention. It happens when the conditions in the tissues become so abnormal that the arterioles and capillaries are unable to contract, and so widespread peripheral vasodilation occurs, causing a fatal drop in blood pressure. This event is called circulatory collapse. Blood flow through the capillaries stops and the tissues quickly begin to die by necrosis, causing effects that spread rapidly throughout the body.

PUZZLE GRID

35 t
36 cyanosis
37 o
38 a
39 echocardiogram
40 m
41 d
r
t
n
y
h
g
s
42 gallop
43 v
44 aricosities
i
c
45 p
t
s
o
r
l
a
e
h
t
p
h
46 th
47 rombus
r
e
a
l
y
h
d
r
i
a
t
48 hypertension
i
c
o
i
s
u
a
a
s
c
t
m
r
d
h
49 auscultation
50 m
l
s
c
y
i
m
i
l
d
i
a
51 antihypertensive
52 foamcells
c
r
f
t
r
n
f
a
a
i
e
54 arteriosclerosis
55 murmur
v
s
c
i
r
56 hypoxaemia
t
t
s
y
r
e
i
s
n
o
57 embolism
o
n
s
i
58 anginapectoris

114

6 The respiratory system

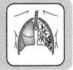

INTRODUCTION

The respiratory system consists of the upper and lower airways, lungs and associated blood vessels.

Disease or trauma to the respiratory system can affect the airway structures, mechanics of breathing, or the nervous and endocrine control of ventilation. Respiratory disorders can often be classified as acute or chronic. Chronic disorders often arise as a complication in patients who are already immune-compromised. Symptoms of many respiratory disorders are similar, such as shortness of breath, cough and wheezing.

Peak expiratory flow rate, chest X-ray, bronchoscopy and tissue specimens are common diagnostic tools used in respiratory investigations.

Treatment of many chronic respiratory disorders aims to alleviate symptoms while preventing the patient's condition from deteriorating further. In acute conditions, the priority is to accurately diagnose the disease or illness and commence appropriate treatment quickly.

Nurses are often responsible for the ventilation of patients in a number of treatment settings such as high dependency units (HDUs) or intensive care units (ICUs), so it is important to be familiar with the disorders and treatment of these respiratory conditions.

Useful resources

Nurses! Test Yourself in Anatomy and Physiology (2nd edition)
Chapter 6

Ross and Wilson's Anatomy and Physiology in Health and Illness (14th edition)
Chapter 10

TRUE OR FALSE?

Are the following statements true or false?

1 Asthma is a chronic disorder of the alveoli.

2 The best advice for patients living with asthma is to avoid potential triggers if possible.

3 Pneumonia is an acute infection of the alveoli.

4 Fungal infection of the lungs is the most common cause of pneumonia.

5 Chronic respiratory disease can increase the risk of developing pneumonia.

6 Atelectasis relates to the passage of fluid or solid particles into the lung.

7 Spontaneous and traumatic pneumothorax present with different signs and symptoms.

8 Respiratory alkalosis is a major complication of chronic obstructive pulmonary disorders.

MULTIPLE CHOICE

Identify one correct answer for each of the following:

9 Emphysema can be classified as which type of respiratory condition?

   a) bronchitis

   b) chronic obstructive pulmonary disorder

   c) pneumonia

   d) respiratory failure

10 What is the main risk factor for chronic obstructive pulmonary disorder?

   a) smoking

   b) environmental exposure to toxins

   c) family history

   d) frequent respiratory infections

11 Which of the following is *not* a symptom of asthma?

   a) cough

   b) wheezing

   c) chest infection

   d) chest tightening

12 Which of the following conditions is the most common cause of pulmonary oedema?

   a) end-stage renal disease

   b) congestive heart disease

   c) chronic liver disease

   d) neoplastic disease

13 Tuberculosis is caused by which type of infectious agent?

a) virus

b) bacteria

c) fungus

d) protozoa

14 Which type of lung cancer has the most rapid growth and metastasis rate?

a) adenocarcinoma

b) small-cell

c) large-cell

d) squamous cell

15 Which of the following conditions is commonly associated with the SARS-CoV-2 virus?

a) croup

b) COVID-19

c) SARS

d) influenza

FILL IN THE BLANKS

Fill in the blanks in each statement using the options in this box.
Not all of them are required, so choose carefully!

> bacterial   right ventricular enlargement   viral
>
> left ventricular failure   pneumothorax   salbutamol
>
> salmeterol   bronchoscopy   spirometry
>
> pneumoconiosis

16 Cor pulmonale is _____ _____ _____ caused by chronic pulmonary hypertension.

17 _____ is a short-acting beta$_2$ agonist, used to treat asthma symptoms.

18 *Streptococcus pneumoniae* is the most common cause of _____ pneumonia.

19 _____ is a common diagnostic tool used in all types of lung cancer.

20 _____ is an accumulation of air in the pleural cavity leading to partial or complete lung collapse.

MATCH THE TERMS

Classify each immune disorder listed below:

    A. **infection**
    B. **degenerative**
    C. **congenital**

21 Acute bronchitis _____

22 Chronic bronchitis _____

23 Cystic fibrosis _____

24 Emphysema _____

PUZZLE GRID

Use the clues and word bank to solve the puzzle.

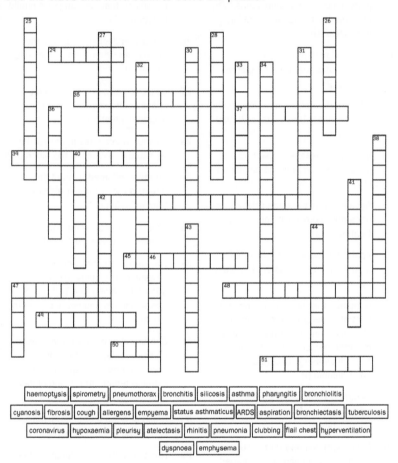

haemoptysis | spirometry | pneumothorax | bronchitis | silicosis | asthma | pharyngitis | bronchiolitis

cyanosis | fibrosis | cough | allergens | empyema | status asthmaticus | ARDS | aspiration | bronchiectasis | tuberculosis

coronavirus | hypoxaemia | pleurisy | atelectasis | rhinitis | pneumonia | clubbing | flail chest | hyperventilation

dyspnoea | emphysema

Clues across

29 Condition marked by acute episodes of spasm in the bronchi of the lungs primarily caused by hypersensitivity reactions that result in breathing difficulties (6)

35 Lung collapse due to the accumulation of air in the pleural space (12)

37 Inflammation of the lung frequently caused by bacterial, viral or fungal infection (9)

39 Infectious disease caused by *Mycobacterium* spp.; consumption (12)

42 Severe sudden asthma attack that does not improve with conventional treatment (6, 11)

45 Abnormal swallowing reflex that may allow foreign material to enter the airways (10)

47 Condition that can be described as central or peripheral, resulting in blue discoloration of the skin and mucous membranes and caused by an increase in deoxygenated haemoglobin (8)

48 Common lower respiratory tract infection that affects babies and young children (13)

49 Pulmonary disease that occurs when the lung becomes damaged and scarred, ultimately resulting in tissue remodelling and loss of elasticity (8)

50 Abbreviated term for respiratory failure characterized by rapid onset of widespread inflammation in the lungs (1, 1, 1, 1)

Clues down

25 Group of related RNA viruses responsible for respiratory conditions that can range from mild to lethal (11)

26 Irritation and inflammation of the mucous membrane inside the nose; coryza (8)

27 Collection of pus in the pleural space commonly caused by bacterial infection (7)

28 Measured decrease in the partial pressure of oxygen in the blood (10)

30 Irritated, inflamed, painful dry throat; a type of upper respiratory tract infection (11)

31 Expectoration of blood from a source below the glottis (11)

32 Long-term condition where the airways of the lungs become widened, leading to a build-up of excess mucus and predisposing to infection (14)

33 Shortness of breath often caused by participation in strenuous exercise, obesity, exposure to extreme temperatures and higher altitudes (8)

34 Rapid or deep breathing, usually caused by anxiety or panic (16)

36 Normally harmless substance that may cause an inappropriate immune reaction and inflammatory response in susceptible individuals (9)

38 Complete or partial collapse of the entire lung or lobule; common respiratory complication following surgery (11)

Clues across (continued)

51 Type of chronic obstructive pulmonary disease caused by a reduction in normally elastic alveolar tissue (9)

Clues down (continued)

40 Changes to the nailbeds that may result from the chronic low blood oxygen levels associated with cystic fibrosis, congenital cyanotic heart disease and other diseases (8)

41 Acute or chronic inflammation of the lining (epithelium) of the bronchi together with a frequent cough and wheezing (10)

42 Interstitial lung disease causing pulmonary fibrosis as a result of prolonged silica exposure (9)

43 Trauma in which broken ribs are isolated from, and interfere with, normal chest movements (5, 5)

44 Term that relates to the basic lung function tests (10)

46 Inflammation of the serous membranes of the lung, usually resulting from viral or bacterial infection (8)

47 Reflex action that initiates to clear the airways of mucus and irritants (5)

ANSWERS

TRUE OR FALSE?

1 | **Asthma is a chronic disorder of the alveoli.**

Asthma is a chronic disorder of the bronchi. During an acute episode, airflow in and out of the lungs is impaired due to narrowing and obstruction of the airways caused by bronchospasm (narrowing of the bronchi when the smooth muscle contracts). Together with irritation, bronchospasm triggers increased mucus secretions and oedema of the mucosa.

2 | **The best advice for patients living with asthma is to avoid potential triggers if possible.**

Knowing and avoiding triggers is most important with all COPD conditions. The main pharmacological (drug) treatment for the relief of asthma symptoms is the beta$_2$-adrenoceptor agonists (or beta$_2$ agonists), which act as bronchodilators by mimicking the action of adrenaline (epinephrine); they can be short-acting or longer-acting. Short-acting treatments, such as salbutamol, work within 5 minutes of administration to relieve symptoms by relaxing the airway muscles and decreasing the mucus secretion for 3–6 hours. Patients who have mild, intermittent asthma symptoms are advised to avoid triggers and would be prescribed beta$_2$ agonists to be taken when they experience symptoms. People who suffer from more frequent symptoms would be prescribed inhaled corticosteroids (steroids) to prevent symptoms, the dose and type of corticosteroid being determined by the severity of symptoms. Patients would also be prescribed a beta$_2$ agonist to relieve symptoms when they occur.

3 | **Pneumonia is an acute infection of the alveoli.**

Pneumonia is an acute infection of the alveoli that impairs gas exchange. It occurs when the protective processes fail to prevent inhaled or blood-borne microbes entering and colonizing the lungs. Prognosis is good for patients with normal lung function and an adequate immune system, but bacterial pneumonia is the leading cause of death in debilitated patients.

4 **Fungal infection of the lungs is the most common cause of pneumonia.**

Bacteria and viruses are the most common cause of pneumonia. Fungal pneumonia is relatively uncommon but may occur in individuals who are immunosuppressed or have immune system disorders such as HIV/AIDS. The pathophysiology of pneumonia caused by fungi is similar to that of bacterial and viral pneumonia.

5 **Chronic respiratory disease can increase the risk of developing pneumonia.**

There are several predisposing factors that can increase the risk of developing bacterial and viral pneumonia such as chronic debilitating illness, lung cancer, cystic fibrosis, smoking or malnutrition. Premature babies are also at greater risk of developing pneumonia due to the under-developed state of their lungs at birth. Aspiration pneumonia is a risk for patients who are debilitated, unconscious or receiving food through a nasogastric tube.

6 **Atelectasis relates to the passage of fluid or solid particles into the lung.**

Atelectasis is the collapse of lung tissue due to compression, absorption or surfactant impairment. Compression atelectasis is caused by external pressure exerted on lung tissue as the result of a tumour or by fluid or air in the pleural cavity. Abdominal distention may cause the alveoli in the lower lung to collapse. Absorption atelectasis often results from the absorption of air from obstructed or hyperventilated alveoli or from the inhalation of pressurized oxygen. Surfactant impairment may cause the lungs to collapse during expiration due to increased surface tension and is commonly associated with prematurity, acute respiratory distress syndrome (ARDS), mechanical ventilation or anaesthesia.

Clinical manifestations of atelectasis are similar to those of pulmonary infection and include dyspnoea, cough, fever and leukocytosis.

7 **Spontaneous and traumatic pneumothorax present with different signs and symptoms.**

Although the causes of each type are quite different, they exhibit similar symptoms, which include a sudden sharp chest pain, exacerbated by breathing and coughing, shortness of breath, cyanosis and respiratory distress. Tension pneumothorax is a dangerous complication that can develop when air is unable to escape from the thoracic cavity, causing pressure to increase around the heart and its major blood vessels. Tension pneumothorax causes severe symptoms such as hypotension, decreased cardiac output, tachycardia and cardiac arrest, and should be treated as a medical emergency.

8 **Respiratory alkalosis is a major complication of chronic obstructive pulmonary disorders.**

Respiratory alkalosis occurs with conditions that are associated with hyperventilation and decreased plasma carbon dioxide (hypercapnia). Stimulation of hyperventilation may be induced by hypoxaemia resulting from pulmonary disease, congestive heart failure, high altitudes, improper use of ventilators, and some hypermetabolic states. In contrast, respiratory acidosis can be caused by diseases or conditions that affect gas exchange in the lungs, such as emphysema, chronic bronchitis, asthma or severe pneumonia. Blockage of the airways (due to swelling or by a foreign object) impairs gas exchange, which can lead to an accumulation of acidic carbon dioxide in the blood. This can induce respiratory acidosis because the blood pH becomes more acidic (drops below pH 7.35). Respiratory acidosis can also be caused by an abnormal control of breathing from the respiratory control centre in the medulla oblongata of the brain (perhaps due to a head injury or stroke). The main symptom is slow, difficult breathing, which may be accompanied by headache, but drowsiness, restlessness, tremor and confusion may also occur. A rapid heart rate, changes in blood pressure and swelling of blood vessels in the eyes may be observed, and the patient may appear cyanosed (blue/purple in colour) due to hypoxia (lack of oxygen). Respiratory acidosis is diagnosed from arterial blood gas (ABG) readings, indicating high carbon dioxide levels. The underlying condition should be treated but patients may be given oxygen therapy and bronchodilators to ease breathing. If untreated, severe cases of respiratory acidosis can lead to coma and death.

 MULTIPLE CHOICE

Correct answers identified in ***bold italics***

9 **Emphysema can be classified as which type of respiratory condition?**

a) bronchitis   ***b)   chronic obstructive pulmonary disorder***
c) pneumonia   d)   respiratory failure

Chronic obstructive pulmonary disorder (COPD) is the classification for chronic, long-term, respiratory disorders that are characterized by obstruction of the airways. Emphysema and chronic bronchitis are also types of COPD. Pneumonia is an acute infection of the lungs that affects gas exchange. In respiratory failure, the lungs cannot obtain enough oxygen (or eliminate sufficient carbon dioxide), which results in the body tissues being starved of oxygen (tissue hypoxia) and being overcome by an accumulation of carbon dioxide (hypercapnia). COPD patients are at risk of acute respiratory failure if their arterial blood gas values deteriorate.

10 **What is the main risk factor for chronic obstructive pulmonary disorder?**

a) *smoking*   b)   environmental exposure to toxins
c)   family history   d)   frequent respiratory infections

Smoking impairs the action and destroys the cilia of the epithelial cells that line the respiratory tract. It also damages the immune action of the macrophages. Together these trigger inflammation of the airways, which increases mucus production, causing alveolar dysfunction and fibrosis (scarring) of the bronchioles. Exposure to environmental toxins such as asbestos, family history and recurring respiratory infections are also risk factors for COPD.

11 **Which of the following is *not* a symptom of asthma?**

a)   cough   b)   wheezing
c) *chest infection*   d)   chest tightening

Cough, wheezing, chest tightening and difficulty breathing are symptoms of asthma. Symptoms depend on the severity of the patient's asthma:

- The least severe form of the disease is mild and intermittent; these patients are symptom-free between attacks.
- An individual who experiences symptoms a few times a week is classified as having mild persistent asthma.
- Patients who experience symptoms daily and have normal or below normal air exchange have moderate, persistent asthma.
- Those with severe persistent asthma experience symptoms continuously and have below normal air exchange. The physical activity of such patients is compromised by their severe symptoms. Chest infections (such as pneumonia) may develop as a complication of asthma. Patients with underlying respiratory

conditions may require hospital treatment such as IV fluids, antibiotics and oxygen therapy, if they develop complications.

12 **Which of the following conditions is the most common cause of pulmonary oedema?**

a) end-stage renal disease   ***b)*** ***congestive heart disease***
c) chronic liver disease   d) neoplastic disease

Pulmonary oedema is defined as an excess of water in the lung. While each of these conditions may be associated in one way or other with pulmonary oedema, it is most commonly associated with congestive heart disease (CHD). Adequate lymphatic drainage, interaction of hydrostatic and oncotic pressures, and capillary permeability ensure the lung normally contains relatively little fluid. Fluid build-up in the lung due to CHD usually results from left ventricular failure, causing pressure on the left side of the heart, together with an increase in pulmonary hydrostatic pressure. When the hydrostatic pressure exceeds the oncotic pressure, fluid eventually moves out of the capillaries and into the lung, leading to oedema.

Pulmonary oedema is now more commonly recognized as a complication of end-stage renal disease due to the increased use of dialysis and survival of these patients. Pulmonary oedema has been reported in some patients with liver disease; its presence increases mortality and the need for liver transplantation. While it may not be directly associated with all forms of neoplastic disease, pulmonary oedema may exist as a frequent complication of cancer treatment that may be cardiogenic or non-cardiogenic in origin.

13 **Tuberculosis is caused by which type of infective agent?**

a) virus   ***b)*** ***bacteria***   c) fungus   d) protozoa

Tuberculosis (TB) is an infection caused by the bacteria *Mycobacterium tuberculosis*. It is an acid-fast organism that usually affects the lungs but may affect other body systems. The disease represents the leading cause of death from curable infections and has recently seen a marked increase in incidence due to disruption of access to essential TB services resulting from the COVID-19 pandemic. The disease is highly contagious and is transmitted through airborne droplets. In susceptible individuals, the bacteria lodge in the peripheral regions of the lung and once inspired into the lower regions, proliferate and cause non-specific pneumonitis. Some bacilli migrate through the lymphatics where they encounter lymphocytes and invoke an immune response. Inflammation in the lung causes neutrophil and macrophage infiltration in an effort to control the spread of infection. However, the bacteria can survive within macrophages and multiply within the cell. Neutrophils, lymphocytes and macrophages isolate the colonies of bacteria, forming a granulomatous *tubercule*. Infected tissues within the tubercule degrade through caseous necrosis, which is then surrounded by collagenous scar tissue preventing further multiplication of bacteria.

Once the bacteria are isolated and immunity develops, TB may remain dormant for life. However, if the immune system becomes compromised or live bacteria escape into the bronchi, active disease can occur through blood and lymphatic spread to other organs. Viruses, fungi, and to a lesser extent protozoa are all capable of causing other respiratory diseases that frequently give cause for concern in the immune-compromised or elderly patient.

14 **Which type of lung cancer has the most rapid growth and metastasis rate?**

a) adenocarcinoma **b) small-cell**
c) large-cell d) squamous cell

Small-cell lung cancer (SCLC) grows most rapidly and metastasizes very early, yet it responds very well to chemotherapy treatment. Unfortunately, any response is relatively short due to the very rapid growth and potential for metastasis of SCLC. Large-cell lung cancer is also rapid growing and metastasis occurs quite early on in disease development (but not as rapidly as in SCLC). Adenocarcinoma is the most common type of lung cancer. It is a moderate-growing lung cancer but with quite early metastasis. The slowest growing type of lung cancer is squamous cell tumours, which are also quite slow to metastasize.

15 **Which of the following conditions is commonly associated with the SARS-CoV-2 virus?**

a) croup **b) COVID-19** c) SARS d) influenza

SARS-CoV-2 is a virus belonging to the severe acute respiratory syndrome-related coronavirus group and is responsible for the COVID-19 pandemic. It is closely related to the SARS-CoV-1 virus responsible for the 2002-2004 SARS outbreak. SARS-CoV-2 infection is characterized by variable symptoms that may include fever, cough, headache, fatigue, distressed breathing, ageusia (loss of taste) and anosmia (loss of smell). Current available evidence indicates that it is most likely of zoonotic origin. The virus shows little genetic diversity, indicating that the transition event introducing SARS-CoV-2 to humans is likely to have occurred in late 2019.

Influenza is a contagious respiratory illness caused by influenza viruses that infect the nose, throat and sometimes the lungs. It can cause mild to severe illness, and at times can lead to death. Croup is a common childhood illness and is most often caused by a parainfluenza virus, although other viruses may be involved. It is characterized by breathing difficulties and a distressing cough and is most active in the winter months. The condition frequently targets children under age 5.

 FILL IN THE BLANKS

16   **Cor pulmonale is *right* *ventricular* *enlargement* caused by chronic pulmonary hypertension.**
Cor pulmonale is a condition that causes the right side of the heart to fail. Long-term high blood pressure in the arteries of the lung and right ventricle of the heart can lead to cor pulmonale. Lung conditions that cause a low blood oxygen level in the blood over a long time can also lead to the condition and include COPD, interstitial lung disease, cystic fibrosis, obstructive sleep apnoea and severe bronchiectasis. Symptoms are variable and may involve cyanosis, chest discomfort and pain, syncope and swelling of the feet or ankles.

17   ***Salbutamol* is a short-acting beta$_2$ agonist, used to treat asthma symptoms.**
Salbutamol is a short-acting beta$_2$ agonist that mimics the action of the natural hormone adrenaline by causing bronchodilation. Longer-acting beta$_2$ agonists are usually administered following treatment with a short-acting drug. They treat symptoms in the same way as short-acting drugs but take around 30 minutes to act and effects last up to 12 hours. Salmeterol is a long-acting beta$_2$ agonist. In addition to beta$_2$ agonist treatment, patients with moderate/persistent symptoms may be prescribed inhaled corticosteroids (hydrocortisone or methylprednisolone), which have anti-inflammatory effects as well as causing bronchodilation as part of the long-term control of asthma.

18   *Streptococcus pneumoniae* **is the most common cause of** *bacterial* **pneumonia.**

These bacteria invade the lungs and settle in the alveoli where they cause an immune response that induces pneumonia symptoms, namely, fever, chills, shortness of breath and fatigue (common in bacterial and fungal pneumonia). Complications arise when bacteria enter the blood from the infected lung, causing serious or even fatal illness such as septic shock.

19   *Bronchoscopy* **is a common diagnostic tool used in all types of lung cancer.**

Bronchoscopy is used to identify the tumour site and often to retrieve tissue specimens for histological examination. Needle biopsy is often used to locate tumours in the peripheral regions of the lungs and to collect tissue for analysis. Chest X-ray is used to locate an advanced lesion, while bone and CT scans are often performed to investigate for metastases.

20   *Pneumothorax* **is an accumulation of air in the pleural cavity, leading to partial or complete lung collapse.**

Pneumothorax can be classified as spontaneous or traumatic. It is usually diagnosed by chest X-ray. Spontaneous pneumothorax most often occurs in patients with chronic pulmonary disorders and in young men (and is often sports-related). Traumatic pneumothorax can have a number of causes such as crushing trauma to the chest (perhaps causing broken ribs), penetrating wound (stabbing, gunshot) and during surgical procedures. If venous return is impeded, a serious complication can develop known as tension pneumothorax (see Answer 7). A small pneumothorax usually clears without treatment over a few days as the body heals the leak and the air is gradually absorbed. For a larger pneumothorax, the air must be removed to relieve symptoms either with a syringe and needle or by inserting a chest drain (placing a drainage tube into the space to allow the air to escape), which may need to remain in place until the lung heals. With a tension pneumothorax, immediate medical treatment is required to relieve the life-threatening symptoms; the air is released by putting a large bore hollow needle directly into the chest.

MATCH THE TERMS

21 Acute bronchitis   **A. infection**

- *Pathophysiology*: Bronchitis is an inflammation of the bronchi that results in an over-production of mucus causing frequent coughing.
- *Causes*: Acute bronchitis can be caused by a bacterial or viral infection but viral infections (usually the same viruses that cause colds and influenza) spread by coughing and sneezing are most common.
- *Risk factors*: Anyone can develop bronchitis, although it can occur with a cold or influenza and is linked with exposure to damp environments.
- *Symptoms*: Productive cough (the cough expels mucus) is the main symptom, but it may be accompanied by wheezing, tightness in the chest and other flu-like symptoms.
- *Diagnosis and treatment*: Many cases of acute bronchitis will clear on their own within a few weeks (described as self-limiting). A diagnosis is made by listening to the chest and considering the symptoms. Treatment is similar to that for a cold or mild influenza, namely, rest and plenty of fluids (to thin out the mucus in the lungs and prevent dehydration). Paracetamol or ibuprofen can be prescribed for aches and pains. Patients are advised to consult a GP if they have an underlying heart or lung condition. An antibiotic will not normally be prescribed (because acute bronchitis is usually caused by viral infection) but if a patient is at risk of pneumonia, a prophylactic (preventative) antibiotic may be recommended.
- *Complications*: Repeated episodes of acute bronchitis can cause permanent damage to the airways, resulting in chronic bronchitis.

22 Chronic bronchitis   **B. degenerative**

- *Pathophysiology*: Chronic bronchitis is a form of COPD characterized by inflammation of the bronchi, which stimulates the over-production of mucus causing frequent coughing. Chronic bronchitis is degenerative because, over time, the persistent coughing causes increasing amounts of mucus to be produced which block the bronchioles and permanently damage the airways. Chronic bronchitis is defined as bronchitis lasting for 3 months or more in the year, over two consecutive years.

- *Causes*: One of the main causes of chronic bronchitis is smoking but it can be caused by other irritants such as chemical vapours.
- *Risk factors*: Patients who experience recurrent respiratory infections are at increased risk.
- *Symptoms*: These are generally the same as with acute bronchitis but chronic bronchitis is persistent and not self-limiting. Chronic bronchitis patients may develop the typical 'blue bloater' symptoms, as the skin appears blue around the lips (cyanosed) due to hypoxia (lack of oxygen) and is bloated due to fluid retention.
- *Diagnosis and treatment*: If the cough persists for more than 3 months in one year and the symptoms recur the following year, chronic bronchitis will usually be diagnosed based on the patient's history. Tests may be conducted to exclude other respiratory conditions (such as pneumonia or lung cancer). The best advice is to cease smoking (where applicable). Patients may be prescribed beta$_2$ agonists to stimulate bronchodilation and corticosteroids to reduce inflammation and ease breathing.
- *Complications*: Patients with chronic bronchitis are more at risk of other respiratory illnesses such as pneumonia or may develop respiratory acidosis (see Answer 8).

| 23 | Cystic fibrosis | **C. congenital** |

- *Pathophysiology*: Cystic fibrosis (CF) is a congenital disease that affects the mucous glands and cells in the body, causing them to secrete excess mucus. These glands and cells are found in the respiratory, digestive and reproductive tracts. The excess mucus in the respiratory tract blocks the airways and causes frequent bacterial infections.
- *Causes*: It is caused by a faulty recessive gene that normally controls salt and water movement in and out of cells. When this gene is faulty, the cells and glands that normally secrete lubricating mucus, instead secrete excess salt (in the form of chloride ions) and not enough water, making mucus secretions thick and glue-like.
- *Risk factors*: There is no way of preventing CF if you have two copies of the recessive gene. CF patients are at greater risk of

recurrent respiratory infections. Families who are known to carry the gene can undergo genetic testing to determine if they are carriers.

- *Symptoms*: Patients have symptoms that affect several of the organ systems associated with the excess mucus that is secreted. Symptoms include recurrent respiratory infections, digestive problems and infertility.

- *Diagnosis and treatment*: Diagnosis is by screening. In the UK, neonates are automatically screened as part of the heel prick test (which also screens for sickle cell anaemia and phenylketonuria, or PKU). There is no cure for CF and it is life-limiting (patients seldom survive beyond their mid-thirties).Treatment is focused on alleviating symptoms: for respiratory symptoms, patients are prescribed bronchodilators and steroids to reduce inflammation and ease breathing. They may also be given an enzyme (DNase) to thin mucus. To aid digestion, patients are given pancreatic enzymes together with vitamin and nutritional supplements. Daily physiotherapy is required to clear the airways and help prevent respiratory tract infections. A lung transplant may be recommended if a patient suffers from respiratory failure and while this does not cure the disorder (because the defective gene is still present), it can relieve respiratory symptoms giving patients improved quality of life for several years.

- *Complications*: CF patients are at high risk of severe respiratory infections such as pneumonia. There is also a high risk of heart and lung failure.

24 Emphysema **D. degenerative**

- *Pathophysiology*: Emphysema is another form of COPD, and is a degenerative condition characterized by progressive shortness of breath due to chronic inflammation, which damages the bronchioles and elasticity of the alveoli, impairing gas exchange. This damage is permanent and irreversible.

- *Causes*: Emphysema is caused by inhaled particles such as smoke or other irritants (e.g. hay or dust) that damage the alveolar membranes. Initially, the lungs can compensate for the affected area using other areas of the lungs so that gas exchange remains efficient, and no symptoms are noticed. However, as the condition progresses and the area of gas exchange is reduced, the patient will begin to experience symptoms (particularly upon exertion). In rare cases, emphysema is caused by a deficiency in the enzyme alpha 1-antitrypsin, which damages the elasticity of the alveoli.

- *Risk factors*: Exposure to cigarette smoking is the biggest risk factor, although certain occupations also carry a hazard, such as those that involve exposure to fumes or dust.

- *Symptoms*: Shortness of breath that gets progressively worse. This may be accompanied by a chronic cough and unintended weight loss as the patient expends more energy by breathing deeper to inhale sufficient oxygen. As the condition progresses, the patient may develop the characteristics of the 'pink puffer' – displaying a reddened complexion due to the effort required in breathing and hyperventilating in an attempt to inhale sufficient oxygen. They may also develop a characteristic expanded 'barrel chest' as the thoracic cage expands due to increased compliance in the lungs.

- *Diagnosis and treatment*: Like chronic bronchitis (another form of COPD), diagnosis is based on the patient's history. There will be a progressive deterioration in lung function tests (such as spirometer readings) and in arterial blood gas (ABG) values. Further tests may be conducted to eliminate other possible respiratory disorders. The best advice is to cease smoking (where applicable). Patients may be prescribed beta$_2$ agonists to stimulate bronchodilation and corticosteroids to reduce inflammation and ease breathing.

- *Complications*: As with chronic bronchitis, emphysema patients are more at risk of other respiratory illnesses such as pneumonia or may develop respiratory acidosis (see Answer 8).

PUZZLE GRID

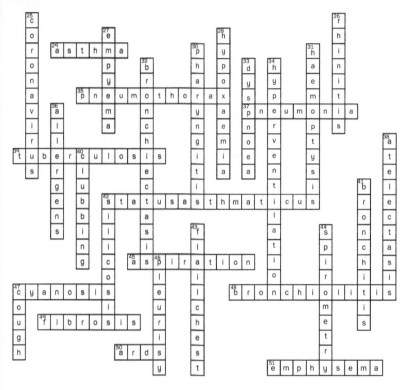

7 The urinary system

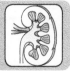

INTRODUCTION

The urinary (renal) system consists of the kidneys (which produce urine) and ureters, bladder and urethra (which store and transport urine before urination). The main function of this system is the filtration of blood and collection and excretion of waste products. Other vital roles of the kidneys include maintaining the acid–base balance of the blood, regulating intracellular and extracellular fluid balance, and maintenance of blood pressure.

Disorders of the urinary system can be life-threatening if left untreated. Many of the symptoms of early disease are non-specific and include fatigue, lethargy, altered blood pressure, nausea and vomiting. Often it is only after certain blood tests, such as for creatinine clearance rate, that renal problems become apparent. Specific symptoms include pain and change in frequency of urination. The location and nature of the pain usually indicate the source of the problem.

It is important that such diagnostic tests are performed promptly and accurately interpreted so that the necessary interventions can be made quickly, since some renal disorders can deteriorate very rapidly. Many disorders are associated with fluid imbalance and can be directly related to renal problems, or are secondary to a disorder of another organ system. These are commonly encountered by nurses in a variety of treatment settings, so it is essential to have a thorough understanding of the urinary system and its associated functions.

Useful resources

Nurses! Test Yourself in Anatomy and Physiology (2nd edition)
Chapter 7

Ross and Wilson's Anatomy and Physiology in Health and Illness (14th edition)
Chapter 13

Fluids and Electrolytes Made Incredibly Easy (1st edition)

TRUE OR FALSE?

Are the following statements true or false?

1   Irreversible destruction of renal tissue occurs in chronic kidney disease.

2   A pathophysiological sign of chronic kidney disease is an imbalance of fluids and electrolytes.

3   Acute renal failure occurs when there is a sudden interruption of renal function, usually due to an obstruction.

4   Serum creatinine levels are a good diagnostic indicator of early acute renal failure.

5   Kidney stones develop when substances that normally dissolve in the urine form hard crystals.

6   Metabolic acidosis can occur due to excessive loss of bicarbonate ions from severe, prolonged diarrhoea.

7   Administering sodium chloride is the best treatment option for acute metabolic acidosis when blood pH is < 7.1.

8   Cystitis is an infection of the upper urinary tract.

a b
c d   **MULTIPLE CHOICE**

Identify one correct answer for each of the following:

9 Chronic kidney disease occurs in how many stages?

a) 2

b) 3

c) 4

d) 5

10 Which of the following is *not* a classification of acute renal failure?

a) interrenal failure

b) intrarenal failure

c) postrenal failure

d) prerenal failure

11 Treatment of acute renal failure does *not* include which of the following?

a) administration of protein, sodium and potassium supplements

b) fluid restriction

c) high-calorie diet

d) monitoring fluid and electrolyte balance

12 Which of the following is the most accurate measurement of the glomerular filtration rate?

a) blood pressure

b) blood urea nitrogen

c) creatinine clearance

d) urine output volume

13 Metabolic alkalosis is characterized by:

a) a decrease in bicarbonate ions

b) an increase in bicarbonate ions

c) decreased blood pH

d) an increase in hydrogen ions

14 Which of the following is *not* a cause of metabolic acidosis?

a) diabetic ketoacidosis

b) excessive ingestion of alkali

c) inefficient excretion of hydrogen ions

d) severe diarrhoea

15 The main treatment for a lower urinary tract infection is:

a) antibiotics

b) IV fluids

c) painkillers

d) rest and fluids

16 Which of the following serum bicarbonate (HCO_3^-) values would indicate a patient is suffering from metabolic acidosis?

e) < 22 mmol/L

f) > 22 mmol/L

g) < 26 mmol/L

h) > 26 mmol/L

17 The most common form of treatment for larger kidney stones is:

a) extracorporeal shock wave lithotripsy

b) percutaneous nephrolithotomy

c) traditional surgery

d) ureteroscopy

18 Which of the following is *not* a symptom of glomerulonephritis?

a) frequent urination

b) haematuria

c) kidney pain

d) proteinuria

19 Which of the following is *not* advised in the treatment of glomerulonephritis?

a) avoid alcohol

b) drink plenty of water

c) follow a strict diet

d) limit salt intake

FILL IN THE BLANKS

Fill in the blanks in each statement using the options in this box.
Not all of them are required, so choose carefully!

compensation	urea	bicarbonate
gallstones	ECG	creatinine
amylase	1000 mL/minute	renal colic
100 mL/minute	septicaemia	equilibrium
sodium	dialysis	

20 _____ is a treatment used in cases of kidney failure.

21 Clinical manifestation of acute renal failure is characterized by a sudden increase in serum _____ and _____.

22 Loss of _____ ions can cause metabolic acidosis in chronic kidney disease.

23 The severe pain of kidney stones is sometimes called _____ _____.

24 The normal creatinine clearance level is considered to be _____ or more.

25 To correct abnormal pH, metabolic acidosis may stimulate an opposing abnormality, respiratory alkalosis, which is known as _____.

PUZZLE GRID

Use the word bank and clues below to solve the puzzle.

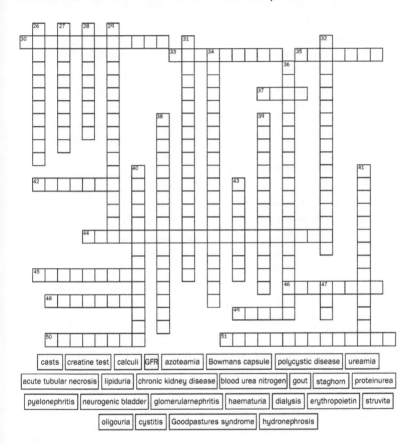

Word bank:

casts | creatine test | calculi | GFR | azoteamia | Bowmans capsule | polycystic disease | ureamia

acute tubular necrosis | lipiduria | chronic kidney disease | blood urea nitrogen | gout | staghorn | proteinurea

pyelonephritis | neurogenic bladder | glomerularnephritis | haematuria | dialysis | erythropoietin | struvite

oligouria | cystitis | Goodpastures syndrome | hydronephrosis

Clues across

30 Diagnostic assay that determines the efficiency of waste removal by the kidneys (8, 4)

33 Marked reduction in urine volume (9)

Clues down

26 Presence of protein in the urine; major sign of kidney disease (11)

27 Presence of blood in the urine (10)

28 Presence of lipid in the urine; frequent sign of nephrotic syndrome (9)

Clues across (continued)

35 Hard deposits made of minerals and salts that form inside the kidneys, resulting in severe pain and potential infection (7)

37 Severe and painful form of arthritis caused by the accumulation of uric acid crystals in the joint space (4)

42 Serious complication of chronic kidney disease and acute kidney injury that occurs when urea fails to be eliminated from the circulation (7)

44 Gradual loss of renal function over time (7, 6, 7)

45 Elevated levels of primary and secondary nitrogenous waste products in blood (9)

46 Complex renal calculi that occupy most of the renal collecting system (8)

48 Inflammation of the bladder usually as a result of a urinary tract infection (8)

49 Microscopic cylindrical structures produced in the kidney and present in the urine in certain disease states (5)

50 Type of kidney stone commonly formed when the urine becomes more alkaline; infection stone (8)

51 Swelling of one or both kidneys due to impaired urinary drainage via the ureters (14)

Clues down (continued)

29 Condition in which problems with the nervous system affect the bladder and urination (10, 7)

31 Inflammation of the renal filtration apparatus often as a result of immune dysfunction (19)

32 Measure of the amount of nitrogen in blood that comes from the waste product urea (5, 4, 8)

34 Rare autoimmune condition affecting lungs and kidneys; anti-GBM disease (12, 8)

36 Severe condition commonly caused by ischaemic or nephrotoxic injury to the epithelial cells of the renal tubes (5, 7, 8)

38 Genetic condition whereby numerous fluid-filled sacs form within the kidneys (10, 7)

39 Essential hormone secreted by the kidneys in response to hypoxia (14)

40 Structural component of the nephron that collects fluids from glomerular blood (7, 7)

41 Urinary tract infection where one or both kidneys become infected, usually with *Escherichia coli* (14)

43 Procedure employed to remove waste products and excess fluid from the blood in situations of renal failure (8)

47 Glomerular filtration rate; overall index of kidney function (1, 1, 1)

ANSWERS

 TRUE OR FALSE?

1 **Irreversible destruction of renal tissue occurs in chronic kidney disease.** ✔

This is accompanied by gradual loss of kidney function. Occasionally, chronic kidney disease (CKD) arises suddenly, damaging the nephrons and resulting in a rapidly progressing disease that causes irreversible kidney damage.

2 **A pathophysiological sign of chronic kidney disease is an imbalance of fluids and electrolytes.** ✔

Clinical features of fluid and electrolyte imbalance include hypervolaemia, hypocalcaemia, hyperkalaemia, hyperphosphataemia, hypertension, irregular heartbeat, fatigue and nausea. Patients with CKD will also experience symptoms such as fatigue, dyspnoea, haematuria, nocturia, itching, oedema and (in males) erectile dysfunction. Chronic kidney disease may develop as a complication of diabetes (types 1 and 2), hypertension and overuse of NSAIDs.

3 **Acute renal failure occurs when there is a sudden interruption of renal function, usually due to an obstruction.** ✔

Kidney obstruction is usually caused by renal calculi (stones). Other causes include hypovolaemia (low blood volume), poor circulation or kidney disease. It is a reversible condition but, if left untreated, it can result in permanent damage and lead to CKD. During hypovolaemia, cells in the kidneys secrete renin that stimulates the production of angiotensin, which causes blood vessels to constrict (vasoconstriction), resulting in increased blood pressure. Angiotensin also stimulates the secretion of aldosterone (vasopressin) from the adrenal cortex, which causes the kidney tubules to increase the reabsorption of sodium and water into the blood. This increases the volume of fluid in the body, which also increases blood pressure.

4 | **Serum creatinine levels are a good diagnostic indicator of early acute renal failure.**

Serum creatinine can remain within the normal range despite the loss of over 50% of renal function, thus measurement of serum creatinine levels is not a good diagnostic test in early-stage acute renal failure.

5 | **Kidney stones develop when substances that normally dissolve in the urine form hard crystals.**

Also known as renal calculi, kidney stones develop when salts or minerals, normally found in urine, form solid crystals inside the kidney. Usually, these crystals are so small they pass harmlessly out of the body unnoticed. However, they can build up, forming a much larger stone that is difficult to pass, causing severe acute pain in the back or side (or occasionally the groin), which may last for minutes or even hours. A small kidney stone (less than 4 mm in diameter) may be collected by filtering the urine though some gauze. For large stones (that will not pass), imaging techniques such as X-ray, CT scan or ultrasound can be used to locate the stone. Another imaging technique called intravenous pyelogram, IVP (or intravenous urogram, IVU), is an X-ray of the urinary system using a contrast medium dye (injected into a vein) that highlights any blockages as the dye is filtered out of the blood by the kidneys. Once the stone is located, treatment and removal options can then be determined.

6 | **Metabolic acidosis can occur due to excessive loss of bicarbonate ions from severe, prolonged diarrhoea.**

Metabolic acidosis is an acid–base imbalance that occurs when the blood is too acidic. Acid is a by-product of the breakdown of fats during digestion. Normally, the body can make bicarbonate ions to neutralize the acids produced in digestion but sometimes the body cannot make enough bicarbonate or too much of it is excreted. A lot of water and electrolytes (including bicarbonate) may be lost from the body during an episode of diarrhoea. It may also be caused by an accumulation of acidic hydrogen ions (H^+) caused by a respiratory disorder that prevents removal of excess CO_2 from the blood – respiratory acidosis (see Chapter 6, Answer 8).

7 | **Administering sodium chloride is the best treatment option for acute metabolic acidosis when blood pH is < 7.1.**

Administering bicarbonate will neutralize the excess hydrogen ions, to treat acute metabolic acidosis. However, it is not normally recommended if the underlying cause of metabolic acidosis is unclear because this can lead to the opposite disorder – metabolic alkalosis. The kidneys help to regulate blood pH by excreting the hydrogen ions in urine and, although this is slow, excretion in urine is the main way to eliminate excess acids from the body, especially in cases of mild metabolic acidosis.

8 **Cystitis is an infection of the upper urinary tract.**
Cystitis is an infection of the bladder, which is part of the lower urinary tract; the other part of the lower urinary tract is the urethra, an infection of which is called urethritis. A urinary tract infection (UTI) develops when part of the urinary tract becomes infected, usually by bacteria. Bacteria usually enter the urinary system through the urethra or, more rarely, through the bloodstream. UTIs are more common in females than males because the female urethra is shorter and closer to the anus than in males, which can allow bacteria from the anus to enter the urinary tract more easily. Symptoms include pain or a burning sensation during urination (dysuria), frequent need to urinate and lower abdominal pain. Infections are usually mild and usually resolve within 4–5 days. Antibiotics can be prescribed to clear the infection and speed up recovery. Some patients experience repeated UTIs, which can be treated with long-term antibiotics to prevent recurrent infections.

MULTIPLE CHOICE

Correct answers identified in **bold italics**

9 **Chronic kidney disease occurs in how many stages?**

a) 2 b) 3 c) 4 **d) 5**

There are five stages of progression in CKD:

Stage 1: Kidney damage with normal or increased GFR ($\geq$ 90 mL/min).
Stage 2: Kidney damage with minor decrease in GFR (60–89 mL/min).
Stage 3: Moderate decrease in GFR (30–59 mL/min).
Stage 4: Severe decrease in GFR (15–29 mL/min).
Stage 5: Kidney failure (< 15 mL/min or dialysis).

10 **Which of the following is *not* a classification of acute renal failure?**

a) ***Interrenal failure***   b) intrarenal failure
c) postrenal failure   d) prerenal failure

Interrenal failure is not a classification of acute renal failure. Prerenal failure develops due to insufficient blood flow to the kidney (hypoperfusion) and may be caused by vasoconstriction, hypotension, hypovolaemia or decreased cardiac output. Prerenal failure can rapidly be reversed by restoring blood flow. Intrarenal failure occurs when damage occurs to the filtration mechanism of the kidney tubules. Postrenal failure is caused by obstruction of urine flow from the kidneys.

11 **Treatment of acute renal failure does *not* include which of the following?**

a) administration of protein, sodium and potassium supplements
b) fluid restriction
c) high-calorie diet
d) monitoring fluid and electrolyte balance

Intake of protein, sodium and potassium should be limited when treating for acute renal failure since levels of these may be elevated during the illness. All other measures should be taken when treating acute renal failure.

12 **Which of the following is the most accurate measurement of the glomerular filtration rate?**

a) blood pressure b) blood urea nitrogen
c) creatinine clearance d) urine output volume

Creatinine is filtered out of the blood by the glomeruli and not reabsorbed by the tubules, so it is an accurate measurement of the filtration rate of the glomeruli. It reflects how much fluid the kidneys have filtered over a 24-hour period. The test involves comparing the amount of creatinine in the blood with the amount excreted in urine over a given period. All urine produced over 24 hours is collected and a blood sample taken to test serum creatinine levels in the blood.

13 **Metabolic alkalosis is characterized by:**

a) a decrease in bicarbonate ions
b) an increase in bicarbonate ions
c) decreased blood pH
d) an increase in hydrogen ions

In metabolic alkalosis, levels of bicarbonate ions in the blood serum increase, which in turn makes the blood more alkaline and increases the blood pH. This suppresses the respiratory centre in the medulla, inhibiting respiration. Levels of carbon dioxide in the blood will increase as the body attempts to correct the blood pH but this compensation by the respiratory system is usually limited. Metabolic alkalosis is the opposite acid–base disorder to metabolic acidosis.

14 **Which of the following is *not* a cause of metabolic acidosis?**

a) diabetic ketoacidosis
b) excessive ingestion of alkali
c) inefficient excretion of hydrogen ions
d) severe diarrhoea

Excessive alkali will increase the blood pH (> pH 7.45) and so can trigger metabolic alkalosis but not metabolic acidosis. The other three situations can lead to development of metabolic acidosis.

15 **The main treatment for a lower urinary tract infection is:**

a) antibiotics	b) IV fluids
c) painkillers	d) rest and fluids

Lower UTIs and mild-to-moderate upper UTIs are usually treated at home with a course of antibiotics for 3–7 days; the length of the course will depend on the severity of symptoms and the risk of developing complications. Painkillers such as paracetamol or ibuprofen may be taken to relieve pain (however, ibuprofen is not recommended during pregnancy). Treatment at home for an upper UTI usually involves taking antibiotics for 7–14 days. Some patients who develop upper UTIs will require hospital admission, namely, diabetics and patients who are immunocompromised. Patients who develop severe upper UTIs and are over the age of 60 or pregnant may also require hospitalization. Hospitalized patients are treated with IV fluids and antibiotics and will have their blood and urine monitored regularly. Patients usually respond well to hospital treatment and are discharged within 7 days.

16 **Which of the following serum bicarbonate (HCO_3^-) values would indicate a patient is suffering from metabolic acidosis?**

a) < 22 mmol/L	b) > 22 mmol/L
c) < 26 mmol/L	d) > 26 mmol/L

The acceptable normal range of blood serum bicarbonate ions (HCO_3^-) is 22–26 mmol/L. When bicarbonate levels fall below

22 mmol/L, the patient is in metabolic acidosis. When bicarbonate levels in the systemic arterial blood exceed 26 mmol/L, the condition is called metabolic alkalosis.

17 | **The most common form of treatment for larger kidney stones is:**

a) *extracorporeal shock wave lithotripsy*
b) percutaneous nephrolithotomy (PCNL)
c) traditional surgery
c) ureteroscopy

Larger stones (> 6 mm in diameter) and stones located in a ureter often require hospital treatment in the form of extracorporeal shock wave lithotripsy (ESWL), percutaneous nephrolithotomy (PCNL), ureteroscopy or traditional surgery. The treatment choice will depend on the size and location of the stone, although the most common method is ESWL, which uses energy waves to break the stone into smaller pieces, which then pass in the urine. ESWL is not suitable for obese patients; they usually undergo the surgical technique, PCNL. If the stone is in the ureter, ureteroscopy (also known as retrograde intrarenal surgery, or RIRS) may be recommended. Traditional surgery is only used in around 5% of cases when no other method is suitable. If the stone is made up of uric acid, patients are advised to drink at least 3 litres of water every day to help dissolve the stone; however, this only works for this type of stone because they are much softer. Complications are rare with kidney stones, although until the blockage is cleared, patients are at increased risk of UTIs (see Answer 8). The most common complication is recurrence of the condition.

18 | **Which of the following is *not* a symptom of glomerulonephritis?**

a) *frequent urination*   b) haematuria
c) kidney pain   d) proteinuria

Glomerulonephritis occurs when the glomeruli (tiny filters in the kidney) become inflamed. This may be due to a bacterial infection or can be secondary to a chronic autoimmune illness (such as systemic lupus erythematosus (SLE); see Chapter 2, Answer 20). When inflamed, the glomeruli do not filter the blood properly, causing an accumulation of salt and excess fluid. Severe glomerulonephritis may prevent urination for 2–3 days. Glomerulonephritis may not cause any obvious symptoms, although small amounts of blood and/or protein may be present in the urine, which may only become apparent upon testing. Not all patients experience kidney pain but when reported, it is important to exclude other conditions such as a UTI or kidney stones. In severe cases of glomerulonephritis, a noticeable amount of blood may be lost through the glomeruli, causing haematuria. If a large amount of protein is lost through the damaged glomeruli in the kidneys, the urine may be cloudy or frothy. The accumulation of fluid can lead to complications such as hypertension and, in some cases, kidney disease or kidney failure can occur.

19 **Which of the following is *not* advised in the treatment of glomerulonephritis?**

a) avoid alcohol   ***b)*** ***drink plenty of water***
c) follow a strict diet   d) limit salt intake

Patients are usually advised to restrict fluid intake and to avoid alcohol, and their diet will have to be carefully controlled, usually under instruction from the GP or dietician, with advice about eating protein and controlling intake of potassium and salt. If the glomerulonephritis is caused by bacteria, an antibiotic will be prescribed and a corticosteroid may also be recommended. If the patient has high blood pressure, an angiotensin-converting enzyme (ACE) inhibitor may also be prescribed to reduce blood pressure and prevent further kidney damage and kidney failure. If the episode is secondary to another illness, it will need to be treated to prevent recurring episodes of glomerulonephritis.

 FILL IN THE BLANKS

20 ***Dialysis*** **is a treatment used in cases of kidney failure.**
If the kidneys fail (such as in end-stage renal failure), an excess of waste products will accumulate in the blood. Dialysis is an artificial method of filtering the blood that mimics the normal functioning kidneys. Without dialysis treatment, kidney failure will be fatal. There are two types of dialysis: haemodialysis and peritoneal dialysis. Dialysis patients must observe a strict diet for their food and fluid intake. The only solution to long-term dialysis is a kidney transplant.

21 | **Clinical manifestation of acute renal failure is characterized by a sudden increase in serum _urea_ and _creatinine_.**

These are the first renal-related symptoms that appear in patients who have previously shown non-specific symptoms. The extent of elevated urea and creatine will depend on the underlying cause and severity of the acute renal failure.

22 | **Loss of _bicarbonate_ ions can cause metabolic acidosis in chronic kidney disease.**

Metabolic acidosis is a symptom of CKD and can be diagnosed from arterial blood gas readings that will indicate a reduced blood pH < 7.35. When normal kidneys excrete excess hydrogen ions from the blood, the tubules reabsorb sodium and bicarbonate ions and return them to the blood. Metabolic acidosis develops because CKD limits excretion of hydrogen ions from the body. The excess hydrogen ions in cells cause the cells to secrete too many potassium, sodium and calcium ions, which causes an overall electrolyte imbalance.

23 | **The severe pain of kidney stones is sometimes called _renal colic_.**

Renal colic is often used to describe the severe pain caused by a stone blocking a ureter. The severe pain is usually located on one or both sides of the back. It is described as sudden, excruciating spasms and is often accompanied with nausea, vomiting, fever, chills, the urine may appear bloody or cloudy, and the patient may experience a frequent need to urinate or a burning sensation when urinating. Similar symptoms indicate a urinary tract infection, so it is important to seek medical advice. Treatment of kidney stones depends on the type of stone: small stones often pass naturally in the urine; patients are usually advised to drink lots of water to encourage urination and keep the urine colourless. Often patients are asked to filter their urine through gauze so they will know when the stone has passed. Patients may be prescribed a painkiller and antiemetic to relieve symptoms. Pain usually subsides a few days after the stone passes.

24 | **The normal creatinine clearance level is considered to be _100_ _mL/minute_ or more.**

A value lower than 100 mL/minute indicates the kidneys are not functioning efficiently enough. Obese patients may not be able to obtain accurate creatinine clearance results. Creatinine clearance rates decrease with age. Blood urea nitrogen (BUN) levels are a measure of the amount of nitrogen in blood as determined by the amount of detectable urea. BUN is a useful indicator of renal function but creatinine clearance is considered more accurate.

25 **To correct abnormal pH, metabolic acidosis may stimulate an opposing abnormality, respiratory alkalosis, which is known as _compensation_.**

Compensation is triggered by the body to try to restore homeostasis of blood pH. There are two mechanisms: (1) respiratory hyperventilation or (2) increasing bicarbonate production (by the kidneys). Hyperventilation can compensate for the decreasing blood pH by exhaling extra carbon dioxide; this raises the blood pH by removing the acid-causing carbon dioxide. Increasing the production of the alkaline bicarbonate compensates for metabolic acidosis by raising the blood pH, thus helping to neutralize the acidic nature of the blood.

PUZZLE GRID

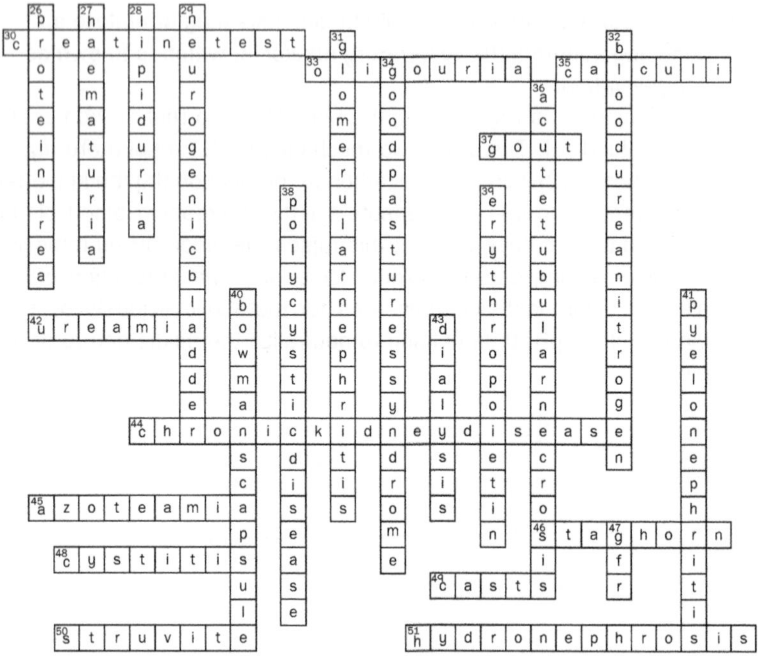

26 proteinurea
27 haematuria
28 lipiduria
29 neurogenicbladde
30 creatinetest
31 glomerularnephritis
32 bloodureanitrogen
33 oligouria
34 goodpasturessyndrome
35 calculi
36 acutetubularnecrosis
37 gout
38 polycysticdisease
39 erythropoietin
40 bowmanscapsule
41 pyelonephritis
42 ureamia
43 dialysis
44 chronickidneydisease
45 azoteamia
46 staghorn
47 gfr
48 cystitis
49 casts
50 struvite
51 hydronephrosis

8 The digestive system

INTRODUCTION

The digestive system, consisting of the gastrointestinal (GI) tract and the accessory digestive organs, is responsible for processing all food and absorbing the nutrients derived from the diet into the blood to supply all the cells, tissues and organs of the body.

Diseases or disorders of any part of the GI tract can produce severe metabolic symptoms that can be life-threatening. An important part of diagnosis is to differentiate between the common disorders and the acutely life-threatening illnesses that often have similar symptoms.

Many of the diagnostic tools for investigative procedures on the GI tract are similar. The suspected location of ulcers or obstructions will determine the tool used. Sigmoidoscopy and colonoscopy can be used to visualize inside the lower regions of the GI tract along with a barium enema, while a barium swallow is used to visualize the upper regions of the GI tract.

Several GI diseases can be prevented by eating a good diet that is low in salt and fat (particularly saturated fat) and high in fibre.

Nurses should know that the GI system is controlled by a range of nervous and hormonal messages and relies on an adequate supply of blood from the cardiovascular system. It is intimately related to these systems, so a thorough understanding of these links is essential when diagnosing, treating and caring for patients with disorders of the GI system.

TRUE OR FALSE?

Are the following statements true or false?

1 The lower oesophageal sphincter prevents the duodenal contents flowing back into the stomach.

2 Obesity is a risk factor for cholecystitis.

3 Liver cirrhosis describes a group of chronic liver diseases.

4 Crohn's disease is a type of inflammatory bowel disease.

5 The most common cause of acute pancreatitis is alcohol abuse.

6 The bacterium *Helicobacter pylori* is the cause of 50% of all peptic ulcers.

7 Anorexia nervosa is a psychogenic condition observed primarily in young women.

8 Colorectal cancer has a slow onset and progression.

9 A hereditary component has been implicated in the aetiology of colorectal cancer.

10 Antiemetic medication is usually prescribed to treat norovirus infections.

MULTIPLE CHOICE

Identify one correct answer for each of the following:

11 Cholecystitis is inflammation of which digestive organ?

a) gall bladder

b) stomach

c) liver

d) pancreas

12 Which of the following is *not* a symptom of Crohn's disease?

a) abdominal pain

b) diarrhoea

c) malaise

d) weight gain

13 Which of the following drugs is *not* used when treating Crohn's disease?

a) corticosteroids

b) opioids

c) anti-diarrhoeal medication

d) paracetamol

14 Symptoms of pancreatitis often start as an abdominal pain located in which region?

a) mid-epigastric region

b) upper right quadrant

c) lower back

d) lower left quadrant

15 Melena is an indication of:

a) upper gastrointestinal bleeding

b) lower gastrointestinal bleeding

c) both

d) neither

16 *Helicobacter pylori*-induced peptic ulcers are usually treated with:

a) NSAIDs

b) antacids

c) paracetamol

d) antibiotics

17 Jaundice is a yellow-greenish pigmentation of the skin caused by:

a) hyperlipidaemia

b) hyperbilirubinaemia

c) hyperinsulinaemia

d) hypercholesterolaemia

18 Which of the following pre-existing conditions is *not* a risk factor for colorectal cancer?

a) colorectal polyps

b) hereditary non-polyposis colorectal cancer

c) Crohn's disease

d) liver cirrhosis

FILL IN THE BLANKS

Fill in the blanks in each statement using the options in this box.
Not all of them are required, so choose carefully!

gallstones	melena	hepatitis
amylase	endoscopy	haematochesia
appendicitis	septicaemia	protease
cirrhosis	norovirus	GORD
coronavirus	pancreatitis	

19 _____ infections are the most common cause of gastroenteritis.

20 Lower intestinal bleeding is often indicated by _____.

21 _____ is a severe complication of cholecystitis that can be life-threatening.

22 Frequent regurgitation of chyme from the stomach to the oesophagus is symptomatic of _____.

23 Elevated _____ and lipase levels indicate pancreatitis.

24 The major diagnostic test for duodenal ulcers is _____.

25 Increasing pain that tends to settle in the lower right side of the abdomen is a major symptom of _____.

PUZZLE GRID

Use the word bank (below) and clues (overleaf) to solve the puzzle.

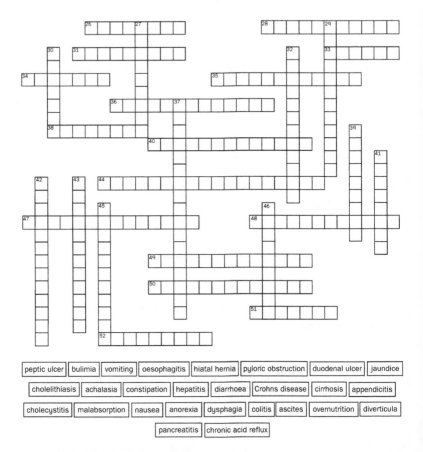

peptic ulcer | bulimia | vomiting | oesophagitis | hiatal hernia | pyloric obstruction | duodenal ulcer | jaundice

cholelithiasis | achalasia | constipation | hepatitis | diarrhoea | Crohns disease | cirrhosis | appendicitis

cholecystitis | malabsorption | nausea | anorexia | dysphagia | colitis | ascites | overnutrition | diverticula

pancreatitis | chronic acid reflux

Clues across

26 Condition in which the skin, sclera and mucous membranes turn yellow because of a high level of bilirubin (8)

28 Sore on the lining of the stomach, small intestine or oesophagus (6, 5)

31 Swallowing disorder involving the oral cavity, pharynx, oesophagus or gastroesophageal junction that may lead to malnutrition, dehydration and aspiration pneumonia (9)

33 Sensation of an urge to vomit that often accompanies infection, food poisoning and motion sickness, among other conditions (6)

34 Inflammation of the large intestine characterized by discomfort and pain (mild and re-occurring over a long period, or acute and severe) in the abdomen (7)

35 Inflammation or swelling of the major accessory organ of digestion that connects to the duodenum (12)

36 Inflammation of the gall bladder caused by trapped bile (13)

38 Eating disorder characterized by low weight, food restriction and body image disturbance (8)

40 Open sore that occurs when the protective mucus lining the wall of the first part of the small intestine breaks down (8, 5)

44 Stenosis of the opening from the stomach into the small intestine (7, 11)

47 Formation of solid deposits in the gall bladder or bile duct; gallstones (14)

Clues down

27 Loose and watery stools that may have an osmotic, secretory or functional aetiology (9)

29 Infrequent or difficult passage of stools that may persist over an extended time (12)

30 Serious, potentially life-threatening eating disorder symptomatic of frequent binge–purge cycles (7)

32 Condition caused by the upper part of the stomach bulging through diaphragm separating the abdomen and chest (6, 6)

37 Persistent backflow of stomach acid into the mouth through the oesophagus often associated with heartburn and acid indigestion (7, 4, 6)

39 Fibrosis of the liver caused by diseases and conditions such as hepatitis and chronic alcoholism (9)

41 Forceful discharge of stomach contents; emesis (8)

42 Type of inflammatory bowel disease that can lead to abdominal pain, severe diarrhoea, fatigue, weight loss and malnutrition (6, 7)

43 Inflammation of the small pouch that projects from the colon on the lower right side of the abdomen (12)

45 Small, bulging pouches that can form in the lining of the digestive system that may become infected and inflamed (11)

46 Inflammation of the liver that may result from a viral infection or liver damage caused by drinking alcohol (9)

Clues across (continued)

48 Condition caused by repeated gastric reflux into the lower oesophagus, producing redness and ulceration (12)

49 Excessive consumption of nutrients and food to the point at which health may be adversely affected (13)

50 Difficulty with the digestion or absorption of nutrients from food that can affect growth and development, or can contribute to specific illnesses (13)

51 Collection of fluid within the abdomen (7)

52 Neurological problem with the oesophagus that makes it difficult to pass solids and liquids into the stomach (9)

TRUE OR FALSE?

1 | The lower oesophageal sphincter prevents the duodenal
contents flowing back into the stomach.
The lower oesophageal sphincter (LOS) prevents the backflow of
stomach contents into the oesophagus. If the sphincter mechanism
fails, gastric reflux (heartburn) may arise (although this is not related
to a cardiac problem). The LOS relaxes during swallowing to allow
food to enter the stomach. When this fails to occur, achalasia may
develop. The main symptoms of achalasia are dysphagia (difficulty
swallowing) and regurgitation of undigested food. A whole meal can
become trapped in the oesophagus, resulting in severe chest pain
that is often confused with heart pain. The pyloric sphincter controls
the release of chyme into the duodenum from the stomach and the
prevention of backflow.

2 | Obesity is a risk factor associated with cholecystitis.
Obesity and a high-cholesterol diet are major risk factors for cholecystitis. Others include high oestrogen levels, diabetes mellitus,
liver disease and pancreatitis. Symptoms of cholecystitis may
develop quickly over a few hours, the main symptom being pain in
the upper abdomen that is usually worse on the right side under the
ribs. The pain may radiate to the back or right shoulder (see Figure
1.1). Patients may also develop nausea, vomiting, fever, indigestion
and flatulence.

3 | Liver cirrhosis describes a group of chronic liver diseases.
Liver cirrhosis is characterized by irreversible destruction and scarring of the hepatic cells of the liver, which are replaced by fibrous
cells. Cirrhosis has many different causes, some of which are
lifestyle-related, such as alcoholism and malnutrition. Other causes
arise as complications of pre-existing diseases such as hepatitis or
right-side heart failure, which causes prolonged venous congestion
in the liver. A liver biopsy will reveal the extent of liver tissue necrosis and fibrosis. A CT scan can also be used to determine liver size,
abnormal masses or obstructions that may be present in the liver,

affecting blood flow through the liver. Blood tests can determine if liver enzymes are elevated.

4 | **Crohn's disease is a type of inflammatory bowel disease.**
The severe inflammation can affect any part of the GI tract and can penetrate all layers of the intestinal wall; it may also involve lymph nodes. Ulcers may form when the inflammation progresses into the peritoneum.

5 | **The most common cause of acute pancreatitis is alcohol abuse.**
Pancreatitis is inflammation of the pancreas. The most common cause of acute pancreatitis is alcohol abuse, which accounts for the majority of cases in patients under 40 years. Gallstones are the second most common cause of acute pancreatitis, although this is more frequent in older patients. Other causes include tumours or cysts of the pancreas, kidney failure, drugs and metabolic or endocrine disorders such as high cholesterol or an overactive thyroid. The main symptom of acute pancreatitis is a sudden onset of severe abdominal pain. Treatment involves supporting the body while it recovers by administering pain relief and supplying nutrients and fluids. With treatment, most patients recover in a few days but repeated episodes can lead to long-term inflammation (chronic pancreatitis). In around 20% of patients, acute pancreatitis can become life-threatening. These patients are at risk of sudden hypotension, septicaemia and multi-organ failure.

6 | **The bacterium *Helicobacter pylori* is the cause of 50% of all peptic ulcers.**
The bacterium *Helicobacter pylori* (*H. pylori*) is the cause of 90% of peptic ulcers. Use of nonsteroidal anti-inflammatory drugs (NSAIDs) (including low-dose aspirin for blood thinning) is another major risk factor. Other predisposing factors include genetic factors, stress or anxiety, and blood type. Blood group A may predispose people to stomach ulcers while blood group O is associated with a predisposition to duodenal ulcers.

7 | **Anorexia nervosa is a psychogenic condition observed primarily in young women.**
Anorexia nervosa is a psychogenic disorder characterized by self-imposed starvation. It primarily affects young adolescent women and is associated with a fear of becoming obese despite progressive

weight loss together with a distorted body image. Body weight may be 15% less than normal for age and height. Menstrual function may be absent in those of reproductive age. As the disease progresses, multiple organ systems are affected. Muscle and fat depletion give the individual an emaciated appearance and increases the risk of osteopenia and osteoporosis. Iron deficiency anaemia promotes fatigue and a low white cell count increases the rate of infection. Key electrolytes (sodium, potassium, magnesium and phosphate) may be depleted, and postural hypotension, bradycardia and sleep disturbances may result. The loss of 25–30% of ideal body weight can lead to death through starvation-induced cardiac failure.

8 | **Colorectal cancer has a slow onset and progression.**
Colorectal cancer has a long latent (asymptomatic) phase and progresses slowly, remaining localized for a long time. Individuals are encouraged to report any persistent changes (6 weeks or more) in bowel habit, such as diarrhoea, constipation or blood in the stools because early detection is key to successful treatment and recovery. Non-specific symptoms include abdominal pain, fatigue, bloating or unexplained weight loss.

9 | **A hereditary component has been implicated in the aetiology of colorectal cancer.**
A small number of colorectal cancers may be caused by inherited gene mutations, including familial adenomatous polyposis (FAP), attenuated FAP (AFAP) and Gardner syndrome, which are caused by inherited changes in the APC tumour suppressor gene that assists in control of cell growth. In those affected with inherited changes in the APC gene, cell growth causes hundreds of polyps to form in the colon. Over time, cancer will nearly always develop in one or more of these polyps.

Lynch syndrome (hereditary non-polyposis colon cancer) comprises another set of gene mutations involved in DNA damage repair. A mutation in one of the DNA repair genes may allow DNA errors to go unfixed and affect growth-regulating genes, leading to the development of cancer. Many other gene mutations have been implicated in the disease process.

Another significant risk factor for colorectal cancer is a diet that is high in fat and low in fibre. This is because movement of digested food through the GI tract is slow in the absence of dietary fibre and moving slowly prolongs the mucosal lining's exposure to the faecal matter, which may release toxins that encourage the cells to mutate. Faecal matter can also be irritating to the lining of the GI tract, causing unnecessary inflammation. A sedentary lifestyle, smoking, alcohol consumption and obesity may also contribute to an increased risk of the disease.

10 **Antiemetic medication is usually prescribed to treat norovirus infections.**

Antiemetics are used to treat vomiting. However, gastroenteritis caused by norovirus infection is not normally treated with antiemetics because vomiting is the body's natural mechanism for expelling the virus (diarrhoea is another method). In severe cases, if a patient becomes severely dehydrated from repeated vomiting, an antiemetic may be recommended. Most patients do not seek medical attention in mild to moderate cases of gastroenteritis; patients are treated at home and advised to rest and drink plenty of water to prevent dehydration. Paracetamol can be taken to reduce fever symptoms. Patients should stay at home for 48 hours after they are symptom-free to prevent the spread of infection. If symptoms persist for more than 3 days or if the patient becomes severely dehydrated, medical attention should be sought. Children and older adults are particularly at risk of becoming dehydrated. Severely dehydrated patients may require hospital admission for IV fluids or a nasogastric tube to replace lost fluids. Although laboratory diagnosis is not normally necessary, norovirus can be diagnosed from a stool sample.

 MULTIPLE CHOICE

Correct answers identified in *bold italics*

11 **Cholecystitis is inflammation of which digestive organ?**

a) gall bladder   b) stomach   c) liver   d) pancreas

Cholecystitis is caused by the formation of gallstones (or calculi), which form when bile and cholesterol harden. Cholecystitis may be acute or chronic. Acute cholecystitis can be triggered by a poor blood supply to the gall bladder, often when a gallstone lodges in the cystic duct, causing the gall bladder to become inflamed and painfully distended. Symptoms include the sudden onset of severe right-side, upper-body pain that is constant and may be accompanied by nausea, vomiting or sweating.

12 **Which of the following is *not* a symptom of Crohn's disease?**

a) abdominal pain
b) diarrhoea
c) malaise
d) *weight gain*

Patients with Crohn's disease usually experience weight loss in addition to the other symptoms listed. Additional symptoms may include blood in the stools, nausea and vomiting. Abdominal pain is usually generalized but is sometimes localized to the lower right quadrant of the abdomen. Crohn's disease is caused by a chronic inflammation of the lining of the GI tract – usually the ileum or colon. The cause is unknown, although it is thought to be a combination of genetic and environmental factors.

13 **Which of the following drugs is *not* used when treating Crohn's disease?**

a) cortical steroids
b) opioids
c) anti-diarrhoeal medication
d) *NSAIDs*

Along with drugs, treating Crohn's disease involves lifestyle changes and sometimes surgery. During acute attacks, it is important to maintain fluid and electrolyte balance. Anti-diarrhoeal drugs (such as loperamide) are prescribed to relieve diarrhoea but are not recommended in patients with significant obstruction. Corticosteroids such as prednisone reduce inflammation, thereby relieving diarrhoea, pain and bleeding. Opioids may be prescribed to alleviate pain and diarrhoea. NSAIDs are not usually prescribed to relieve Crohn's disease as they may induce flare-ups in addition to stomach or intestinal ulcers. Around 80% of patients will have surgery at some point to relieve symptoms or if the bowel becomes perforated or an acute obstruction develops. Surgery to remove the inflamed section of the GI tract relieves symptoms but it does not cure the disease – many patients report several years of remission from symptoms after surgery.

14 **Symptoms of pancreatitis often start as an abdominal pain located in which region?**

a) *mid-epigastric region*
b) upper right quadrant
c) lower back
d) lower left quadrant

For many patients, the only initial symptom of pancreatitis is a pain in this region, centred on the navel, which is not relieved after vomiting. This pain may progress to swelling. In acute pancreatitis, the pain may be localized to the upper left quadrant and radiate to the back (see Figure 1.3). The pain often begins suddenly after eating a meal or drinking alcohol and is relieved when the patient is positioned on the knees and upper chest.

15 **Melena is an indication of:**

a) *upper gastrointestinal bleeding*
b) lower gastrointestinal bleeding
c) both
d) neither

Melena is an indication of upper gastrointestinal bleeding most commonly as a result of peptic ulcer disease. However, any bleeding within the upper gastrointestinal tract or the ascending colon can lead to melena and may include malignant tumours affecting the oesophagus, stomach or small intestine, oesophageal varices, haemorrhagic blood diseases, such as thrombocytopenia and haemophilia, in addition to gastritis, and gastric cancer. Melena may also be a complication of anticoagulant medications, such as warfarin. The condition is indicated by the dark black, tarry stools and strong characteristic odour caused by breakdown of haemoglobin by digestive enzymes and intestinal bacteria.

16 ***Helicobacter pylori*-induced peptic ulcers are usually treated with:**

a) NSAIDs   b) antacids
c) paracetamol   *d)* *antibiotics*

Treatment for *H. pylori* infection usually consists of a 1–2-week course of combination antibiotics along with a proton pump inhibitor (PPI) (such as omeprazole) or H_2-receptor antagonist (such as ranitidine) to reduce acid secretion in the stomach, giving ulcers time to heal. This is called eradication therapy. A combination of (usually three) antibiotics is used in case the bacteria have developed a resistance to antibiotics. The antibiotics normally used are amoxicillin, clarithromycin and metronidazole. These can cause unpleasant (but not normally harmful) side effects such as nausea, vomiting or a metallic taste in the mouth. Patients are tested after the treatment (usually using the urea breath test where CO_2 isotope levels on exhaled breath should be reduced if treatment is successful). Serious complications can develop from peptic ulcers, such as gastric bleeding, gastric obstruction and perforation of the stomach lining, which can lead to peritonitis (inflammation of the abdominal lining).

17 **Jaundice is a yellow-greenish pigmentation of the skin caused by:**

a) hyperlipidaemia   *b)* *hyperbilirubinaemia*

c) hyperinsulinaemia   d) hypercholesterolaemia

Jaundice is an abnormal pigmentation of the skin caused by hyper-bilirubinaemia, which itself can result from extrahepatic obstruction to bile flow due to gallstones, intrahepatic obstruction caused by cirrhosis or hepatitis, or excessive bilirubin production due to excessive haemolysis of red blood cells. Extrahepatic obstructive jaundice occurs if the common bile duct becomes occluded due to gallstone formation or pancreatic oedema. When the bile duct becomes obstructed, bilirubin conjugated by the liver cannot flow into the duodenum and accumulates in the liver before being released into the circulation, ultimately resulting in jaundice. Intrahepatic obstruction involves abnormal hepatocyte function and obstruction of bile canaliculi, allowing elevated levels of bilirubin to enter the circulation. Excessive haemolysis of red blood cells or marked haematoma absorption can also cause a build-up of bilirubin through metabolism of the haem component of erythrocytes and inability of the liver to process the excess bilirubin (non-obstructive jaundice).

18 **Which of the following pre-existing conditions is *not* a risk factor for colorectal cancer?**

a) colorectal polyps

b) hereditary non-polyposis colorectal cancer

c) Crohn's disease

d) *liver cirrhosis*

Crohn's disease and ulcerative colitis are bowel conditions that increase the risk of developing colorectal cancer because of the chronic inflammation of the lining of the GI tract. Colorectal polyps are strongly associated with a predisposition for colorectal cancer – the larger the polyp, the greater the risk. Hereditary non-polyposis colorectal cancer (HNPCC or Lynch syndrome) is a genetic disease associated with a very high risk of developing colorectal cancer as well as other cancers of the digestive tract, and patients should be offered regular screening.

FILL IN THE BLANKS

19 *Norovirus* **infections are the most common cause of gastroenteritis.**

The norovirus family of viruses is the most common cause of gastro-enteritis in the UK. The norovirus infection is sometimes called the 'winter vomiting' disease. It is highly contagious, and the virus can survive for several days in a contaminated area. It is spread through contact with an infected person, infected surfaces and objects, or by consuming contaminated food or water. Norovirus infections occur in all age groups but are particularly common in contained environments such as schools, hospitals and nursing homes. Symptoms of a norovirus infection usually pass (without medical attention) within a few days and include nausea, vomiting, diarrhoea and in some cases a fever, headache, stomach cramps and aching limbs (see Answer 10).

20 **Lower intestinal bleeding is often indicated by** *haematochesia*.

Haematochesia is often caused by lower intestinal bleeding resulting from haemorrhoids or diverticulosis, both of which are relatively benign conditions. However, it can also be caused by colorectal cancer, which is potentially fatal. In newborns, haematochesia may be the result of swallowed maternal blood at the time of delivery but can also be an initial symptom of enterocolitis, a serious condition affecting premature infants. In adolescents and young adults, inflammatory bowel disease, particularly ulcerative colitis, also represents a potential for investigation.

21 *Septicaemia* **is a severe complication of cholecystitis that can be life-threatening.**

If the gall bladder becomes severely infected or gangrenous, it can lead to septicaemia, which can be life-threatening. Other possible complications include perforation of the gall bladder, or a fistula (channel) may form between the gall bladder and digestive tract due to prolonged inflammation.

22 **Frequent regurgitation of chyme from the stomach to the oesophagus is symptomatic of** *GORD*.

GORD (gastro-oesophageal reflux disease) is frequently associated with heartburn, regurgitation of acidic chyme, and upper abdominal pain shortly after eating. Symptoms may be present when there is no acid in the oesophagus. Chest pain may also be experienced and consideration should be given to possible cardiac ischaemic disease. Oedema or decreased oesophageal motility may result in dysphagia. Alcohol or acid-containing foods should be avoided as the may increase discomfort. Laryngitis, asthma and chronic cough may also be associated with acid reflux.

23 | **Elevated _amylase_ and lipase levels indicate pancreatitis.**

Serum amylase and lipase levels will be grossly elevated in acute pancreatitis because the inflamed pancreas over-produces these two enzymes. Patients would be admitted to hospital for further tests and treatment. Further tests include ultrasound or a CT scan to detect an enlarged pancreas. If gallstones are suspected of causing acute pancreatitis, an endoscopic retrograde cholangio-pancreatography (ERCP) may be used to determine the exact location of the gallstone. There are no blood tests for chronic pancreatitis, although the physical state of the pancreas is assessed using the other tests described.

24 | **The major diagnostic test for duodenal ulcers is _endoscopy_.**

Endoscopy is used to confirm the presence of a duodenal ulcer and to differentiate duodenal ulcers from gastric ulcers or carcinomas. Endoscopic evaluation allows visualization of lesions and biopsy. Gastrin levels may be evaluated to identify ulcers associated with gastric carcinomas. Stool and serum antigen tests may be used to detect *H. pylori* infection.

25 | **Increasing pain that tends to settle in the lower right side of the abdomen is a major symptom of _appendicitis_.**

Appendicitis is an inflammation of the appendix, usually due to an infection or obstruction. The major symptom is pain in the abdomen that gets worse over several hours and tends to settle in the lower right side of the abdomen and worsens when pressure is applied to the area. Appendicitis is considered a medical emergency; if left untreated, the appendix can perforate, which can cause life-threatening septicaemia. Appendicitis is usually treated by surgically removing the appendix (appendectomy). It is thought to occur more commonly in people who eat a low-fibre diet.

PUZZLE GRID

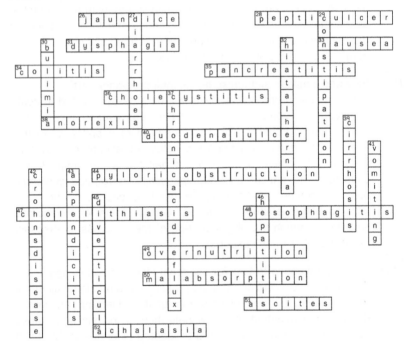

The male and female reproductive systems

INTRODUCTION

Reproduction is a complex process that demands the coordination of a series of anatomical and physiological events. The physiological and anatomical aspects of the reproductive tract are primarily associated with reproduction but there are also psychosocial elements involved in the reproductive process. Dysfunction and disease of any of these components can cause acute and chronic illness, physical and emotional distress, fertility problems, and sometimes even death.

While there are obvious differences in the structure and function of the male and female reproductive systems, several infectious diseases are common to both. Additionally, there exist conditions that are gender-specific and relate to the unique anatomy and physiology of the male and female reproductive systems. These conditions are frequently a result of genetic, endocrine or structural abnormalities that affect reproductive function. Furthermore, several life-threatening malignancies are associated with specific reproductive organs.

Nurses should recognize that the male and female reproductive systems are susceptible to many disorders and that both genders are particularly vulnerable to sexually transmitted infections.

Useful resources

Nurses! Test Yourself in Anatomy and Physiology (2nd edition)
Chapter 12

Ross and Wilson's Anatomy and Physiology in Health and Illness (14th edition)
Chapter 18

Gould's Pathophysiology for the Healthcare Professions (7th edition)
Chapter 19

TRUE OR FALSE?

Are the following statements true or false?

1 Chlamydia infections may be asymptomatic.

2 The most common cause of pelvic inflammatory disease is the human papilloma virus.

3 Polycystic ovary is a condition associated with persistent anovulation.

4 In many cases, prostate cancer will shorten a man's natural lifespan.

5 The incidence of ovarian cancer in Western populations is increasing.

6 Gonorrhoea can present as a localized or systemic infection.

7 Cryptorchidism is associated with an increased risk of testicular cancer.

MULTIPLE CHOICE

Identify one correct answer for each of the following:

8 Which of the following is *not* caused by pre-eclampsia?

a) hypertension

b) hypotension

c) oedema

d) proteinuria

9 The most common site of gonorrhoeal inflammation in males is the:

a) urethra

b) testes

c) prostate gland

d) epididymis

10 The majority of breast tumours are described as:

a) benign

b) malignant

c) ductal

d) lobular

11 Which of the following is *not* a symptom associated with prostate cancer?

a) nocturia

b) hypovolaemia

c) haematuria

d) dysuria

FILL IN THE BLANKS

Fill in the blanks in each statement using the options in this box.
Not all of them are required, so choose carefully!

testicular	gynecomastia	endometriosis
human papilloma	herpes simplex	chlamydia
cervical	ovarian	

12 _____ cancer is linked to sexually transmitted infections.

13 Treatment of _____ may involve manipulation of the normal hormonal cycle.

14 _____ is the overdevelopment of breast tissue in a male.

15 Genital warts are caused by the _____ _____ virus.

16 Prognosis for advanced _____ cancer is quite good.

PUZZLE GRID

Use the word bank (below) and clues (overleaf) to solve the puzzle.

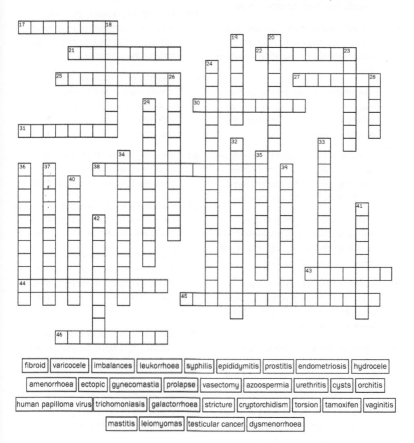

fibroid | varicocele | imbalances | leukorrhoea | syphilis | epididymitis | prostitis | endometriosis | hydrocele

amenorrhoea | ectopic | gynecomastia | prolapse | vasectomy | azoospermia | urethritis | cysts | orchitis

human papilloma virus | trichomoniasis | galactorrhoea | stricture | cryptorchidism | torsion | tamoxifen | vaginitis

mastitis | leiomyomas | testicular cancer | dysmenorrhoea

Clues across

17 Inflammation of one or both testicles most often the result of a sexually transmitted disease (8)

21 Type of swelling in the scrotum that occurs when fluid collects in the tunica vaginalis surrounding a testicle (9)

22 Inflammation of breast tissue that may involve an infection and most commonly affects women who are breastfeeding (8)

25 Defect in the function of the venous valves within the scrotum causing a back-up of blood, enlarged veins and increased scrotal mass (10)

27 Form of pregnancy that occurs when a fertilized egg implants itself outside of the womb, usually in one of the fallopian tubes (7)

30 Painful inflammation that may be associated with a change in colour, odour or abnormal discharge from the birth canal (9)

31 Condition whereby one or more pelvic organs move from their normal location and bulge into the vagina (8)

38 Developmental abnormality in which one or both testes do not move down into their proper place in the scrotum (14)

43 Emergency condition that occurs when a testicle rotates, twisting the spermatic cord that brings blood to the scrotum, often causing severe pain and swelling (7)

Clues down

18 Narrowing of the urethra that slows the flow of urine from the bladder (9)

19 Variable sized non-cancerous growths composed of muscle and fibrous tissue that develop in or around the uterus (7)

20 Surgical procedure for male sterilization or permanent contraception in which the _vasa deferentia_ are cut and tied or cauterized (9)

23 Sexually transmitted disease caused by an infection with the bacteria _Treponema pallidum_ (8)

24 Common group of viruses can cause genital warts or cervical cancer in some individuals; HPV (5, 9, 5)

26 Long-term condition where tissue similar to the lining of the womb starts to grow in other locations, such as the ovaries and fallopian tubes (13)

28 Benign or non-cancerous fluid containing lesions frequently found in the breast or ovaries (5)

29 Nipple discharge unrelated to breastfeeding that may be indicative of an underlying mammary condition (13)

32 Sexually transmitted infection caused by the parasite _Trichomonas vaginalis_ that can cause a foul-smelling vaginal discharge and painful urination in women but is frequently asymptomatic in males (14)

Clues across (continued)

44 Inflammation of the small, coiled tube at the back of the testicle resulting in a swollen, red or warm scrotum together with a gradual build-up of pain (12)

45 Relatively rare but frequently curable neoplasm of the testes (10, 6)

46 Painful and distressing inflammation of the small gland located in the pelvis, between the penis and bladder (9)

Clues down (continued)

33 Period pain caused by certain reproductive disorders, such as endometriosis, adenomyosis or fibroids, or be of idiopathic origin (13)

34 Overdevelopment or enlargement of the breast tissue in males that can occur around puberty (12)

35 Abnormal levels of male hormone that may occur with polycystic ovary syndrome in women of reproductive age (10)

36 Flow of a coloured discharge from the vagina that may be normal or that may be a sign of infection (11)

37 Term used to describe absence of sperm in the ejaculate that may be due to a blockage or defect in sperm production (11)

39 Absence or cessation of menstruation that occurs before menarche, after menopause or in pregnancy, or it may be postoperative if the patient has had a hysterectomy (11)

40 Condition in which the tube that carries urine from the bladder to outside the body becomes inflamed and irritated (10)

41 Anti-oestrogen used to treat oestrogen receptor-positive breast cancer (9)

42 Benign tumour that originates in smooth muscle cells of the myometrium (10)

ANSWERS

TRUE OR FALSE?

1 **Chlamydia infections may be asymptomatic.**

Chlamydia is the most common bacterial infection transmitted through sexual contact. Incidence, particularly in young women, has risen dramatically over the past decade. Most females who have a chlamydia infection of the neck of the womb (cervicitis) have no symptoms (asymptomatic) and do not know that they are infected. In males, infection of the urethra (urethritis) is usually symptomatic, causing a white discharge from the penis with or without pain on urination (dysuria). Occasionally, the condition spreads to the upper genital tract in women (causing pelvic inflammatory disease) or to the epididymis in men (causing epididymitis). If untreated, chlamydia infections can lead to infertility.

2 **The most common cause of pelvic inflammatory disease is the human papilloma virus.**

Pelvic inflammatory disease (PID) is an inflammation of the upper reproductive tract or pelvic cavity that may involve the uterus, the fallopian tubes, the ovaries and the pelvic peritoneum. It is caused by a bacterial infection and can develop if certain sexually transmitted infections (STIs), such as chlamydia or gonorrhoea, remain untreated. Certain procedures such as pelvic operation, postpartum infection, miscarriage or abortion may also increase the risk of developing PID. Individuals may be unaware of symptoms (silent PID) and even when symptoms are present, they can be vague, such as pain in the lower abdomen and pelvis, or deep pain experienced inside the pelvis during intercourse, bleeding between periods and after intercourse, unusual vaginal discharge, fever, vomiting and rectal pain. Most infections occur in sexually active women under the age of 25 and incidence is increasing worldwide. PID has been identified as the leading cause of female infertility. It has also been associated with increasing the risk of ectopic pregnancy. Although the PID infection itself may be cured, effects of the infection may be permanent. This makes early identification essential to reduce the risk of long-term damage to the reproductive system. If the initial infection is mostly in the lower tract, fewer difficulties may be experienced after treatment. If the infection is in the fallopian tubes or ovaries, serious complications are more likely to occur. Treatment generally involves a combination of antibiotics since the infection may be due to multiple bacteria.

3 **Polycystic ovary is a condition associated with persistent anovulation.**

Polycystic ovary (PCO) usually affects females between 15 and 30 years of age. Clinical symptoms may appear after a variable period of normal menstrual function and, in some instances, pregnancy. The symptoms are related to anovulation and include amenorrhoea or dysfunctional bleeding, hirsutism and infertility. A significant number of women with the condition may present as obese. PCO has a spectrum of aetiologies wherein the ovary is affected by the production of excessive amounts of androgens and conversion of these androgens to oestrogens in peripheral tissues prevents ovulation. As well as the symptoms listed above, prolonged anovulation may lead to an increased risk of endometrial cancer, cardiovascular disease and diabetes mellitus.

4 **In many cases, prostate cancer will shorten a man's natural lifespan.** **X**

In many cases, prostate cancer will not affect a man's natural lifespan because it usually progresses very slowly – it can take up to 15 years for the cancer to metastasize (usually to the bones). The cause of prostate cancer remains unknown and the risk of developing the disease increases with age. In the early stages of disease, treatment can cure the cancer although, compared with other cancers, it does not respond well to treatment. Once it has metastasized to the bones, it cannot be cured, and treatment is focused on prolonging life and relieving symptoms. Treatments include removing the prostate, hormone therapy and radiotherapy (using radiation to kill the cancerous cells). All the treatment options carry the risk of significant side effects, including loss of libido, sexual dysfunction and urinary incontinence. For these reasons, many patients opt to delay treatment until there is a significant risk of metastasis.

5 **The incidence of ovarian cancer in Western populations is increasing.**

The incidence of ovarian cancer is increasing in Western populations along with the number of deaths from the disease. Only

25 per cent of ovarian cancers are diagnosed in the early stages, when prognosis is most favourable. There are different types of ovarian cancer, which vary in severity. Genetic factors play a significant role in its development. Early indicators of the disease are vague but should be investigated when they persist. Symptoms are vague and include feeling bloated, indigestion, frequent urination, backache and constipation. The lack of a reliable screening test and non-specific symptoms of the cancer often delay early diagnosis. A large mass may be detected by pelvic examination. Transvaginal ultrasound is the current tool for diagnosis. Treatment involves surgery and chemotherapy; however, the outcome is very dependent on the stage of disease at time of diagnosis.

6 **Gonorrhoea can present as a localized or systemic infection.**
Gonorrhoea is one of the most reported communicable diseases in Western populations. Adolescents and young adults are at higher risk of contracting gonorrhoea with the highest rates among people between the ages of 20 to 24 years. In local gonorrhoea, the symptoms are localized in the reproductive tract, rectum and pharynx. For systemic gonorrhoea, the condition affects major organs in the body, leading to meningitis, polyarthritis, endocarditis, dermatitis and bacteraemia. Vertical transmission of gonococci from an infected mother to the foetus frequently presents as an ocular infection of the newborn that may be difficult to treat. Antibiotic therapy covering penicillin-resistant strains and chlamydial co-infection is recommended for all individuals diagnosed with gonorrhoea together with their partners.

7 **Cryptorchidism is associated with an increased risk of testicular cancer.**
Cryptorchidism is a term describing incomplete testicular descent. Normally, the testes descend into the pelvis by the third month of gestation and then through the inguinal canal into the scrotum during the last 2 months of gestation, thus premature baby boys have a greater risk of being born with undescended testes. Approximately 1% of newborn boys have an undescended testis, a condition which usually resolves within the first year of life. Undescended testes are associated with an increased risk of testicular cancer later in life and may lead to infertility. For these reasons, orchiopexy (the surgical placement of the testis in the scrotal sac) should be performed in cases of persistent cryptorchidism, preferably before 2 years of age, when degenerative tissue changes may begin to develop.

MULTIPLE CHOICE

Correct answers identified in **bold italics**

8 **Which of the following is *not* caused by pre-eclampsia?**

a) hypertension   ***b) hypotension***

c) oedema   d) proteinuria

The causes of pre-eclampsia are not well understood but it is thought to be due to a problem with the blood vessels in the placenta that cause a disruption in the blood supply between mother and baby. The initial symptoms of pre-eclampsia are high blood pressure (hypertension), protein in the urine (proteinuria) and later oedema. If these symptoms develop, they are usually detected at routine ante-natal check-ups. Pre-eclampsia can affect up to 10% of first-time pregnancies, although there is an increased risk if there is a family history or if it occurred in a previous pregnancy. Pre-eclampsia can only be treated by delivering the baby, so until that is possible (from week 37 onwards), patients will be monitored very closely during additional antenatal appointments. In severe cases, the woman may be admitted to hospital. Patients with pre-eclampsia are at risk of developing the more serious condition, eclampsia (convulsions), which can leave the mother permanently disabled or brain-damaged.

9 **The most common site of gonorrhoeal inflammation in males is the:**

a) urethra   b) testes

c) prostate gland   d) epididymis

The most common site of inflammation in males is the urethra, which results in dysuria (painful urination) and a purulent (pus) urethral discharge. The bacteria attach to epithelial cells and damage the mucosa, causing an inflammatory response and formation of pus. Epididymitis may follow, although some males may remain asymptomatic. Gonorrhoea is caused by the bacteria *Neisseria gonorrhoeae*. Many strains of the bacteria have become resistant to treatment with penicillin and tetracycline, making it more difficult to control but ceftriaxone and doxycycline-based therapies may be useful. In females, the infection usually involves the endocervical canal and is frequently asymptomatic, although it may also affect the accessory glands, causing more visible manifestations.

PID usually develops as a serious complication. The newborn may become infected during birth, causing severe eye disease.

10 **The majority of breast tumours are described as:**

a) benign   b) malignant   c) ductal   d) lobular

Up to 90% of tumours discovered in the breasts are benign. All breast lumps discovered by self-examination should be referred to the GP. A patient will probably be referred for a mammogram (X-ray of the breast tissue), although if the woman is under 35, this is unlikely because the breast tissue tends to be denser in this age group, which makes the mammogram less reliable. These patients may be offered an ultra-sound scan instead. A biopsy (usually a needle biopsy) may also be used to diagnose if the cells are malignant. Needle aspiration is used to treat benign cysts by draining fluid from the cyst. When breast tumours are diagnosed as malignant (after a biopsy), patients will usually be referred for further investigation, such as a CT or MRI scan, to determine if the cancer has spread (metastasized). The earlier the diagnosis, the less likely the tumour is to have metastasized. Treatment and outcome will depend on the stage of the cancer.

11 **Which of the following is *not* a symptom associated with prostate cancer?**

a) nocturia   *b) hypovolaemia*
c) haematuria   d) dysuria

Prostate cancer does not normally cause any symptoms until the tumour is large enough to put pressure on the urethra. This results in problems associated with urination such as nocturia, dysuria and, less frequently, haematuria. Symptoms of prostate cancer that is progressing include loss of appetite, weight loss and constant pain. Prostate cancer may be diagnosed from the screening test for prostate-specific antigen (PSA), which detects elevated levels of PSA in the blood. If PSA levels are raised, a digital rectal examination (DRE) will be performed to check for changes to the surface of the prostate gland. If prostate cancer is present, the gland may feel hard and bumpy rather than its normal smooth and firm texture. If there is a possibility that the cancer has metastasized, the patient will be referred for other diagnostic tests, such as a CT or MRI scan, to evaluate the location and extent of metastases. Hypovolaemia describes low blood volume, typically due to a haemorrhage. It can lead to hypovolaemic shock which can be life-threatening.

FILL IN THE BLANKS

12 | *Cervical* **cancer is linked to sexually transmitted infections.**

Cervical cancer is strongly associated with sexually transmitted infections (STIs), particularly herpes simplex type 2 (HSV-2) and certain types of human papilloma virus (HPV). Vaccines against different strains of the virus have recently been developed and should prove effective in reducing the incidence of the malignancy. However, the vaccine is most effective in younger females who are not yet sexually active and so this population has been targeted in the vaccination programme. High-risk factors for cervical cancer include multiple sexual partners, promiscuous partners, sexual contact at a young age and a history of STIs. Preliminary diagnosis via cervical smear is usually confirmed by biopsy, with surgery and radiation being the recommended treatment. The 5-year survival rate is 100% with early diagnosis. Invasive forms of the disease have a less favourable prognosis and depend on the extent of metastases.

13 | **Treatment of** *endometriosis* **may involve manipulation of the normal hormonal cycle.**

Endometriosis is a common condition in which small pieces of the uterine lining (endometrium) are found outside the uterus, such as in the fallopian tubes, ovaries, bladder, bowel, vagina or rectum. Endometriosis commonly causes pain in the lower abdomen, pelvis or lower back. It may also lead to fertility problems. However, some women have few or no symptoms. The cause of endometriosis is uncertain, although it is thought to be hereditary. Treatments do not cure endometriosis but relieve the painful symptoms, either by pain medication, hormonal manipulation or surgery. Hormonal suppression aims to stop the growth of the endometrial tissue while ectopic endometrial tissue can be removed surgically. Depending on the age of the woman, a hysterectomy may be recommended.

14 | *Gynecomastia* **is the overdevelopment of breast tissue in a male.**

Gynecomastia refers to the hyperplastic occurrence of breast tissue in a male. It presents as a firm palpable mass at least 2 cm in diameter located in the subareolar region and may affect up to 40% of the male population. Incidence is greatest among adolescents and men older than 50 years. The condition is caused by hormonal alterations that promote the effect of oestrogen on breast tissues that may result from systemic disorders, drugs, neoplasms or idiopathic aetiologies. All unilateral breast enlargement in males warrants an evaluation for malignancy.

15 **Genital warts are caused by the _human papilloma_ virus.**
Genital warts are caused by an infection with the human papilloma virus (HPV), which is becoming more common. There are many types of HPV that affect the genital tract and some of these have been associated with cervical cancer (see Answer 12). The incubation period for HPV infection may be in excess of 6 months and the disease may be asymptomatic, depending on the location of the lesions. Pregnancy frequently promotes the growth and spread of this highly contagious disease. Genital warts may be removed by a number of different methods, including surgery, laser, cryotherapy and topical caustic agents. Unfortunately, in many cases, they return. The herpes virus is responsible for the occurrence of genital herpes characterized by the appearance of painful ulcerated vesicles (similar to those that appear on the mouth but not caused by the same strain of virus).

16 **Prognosis for advanced _testicular_ cancer is quite good.**
The outlook for testicular cancer is very good because it is one of the most treatable types of cancer. Over 95% of men diagnosed with early-stage testicular cancer will be completely cured. Even advanced testicular cancer, which is where the cancer has spread outside the testicles to nearby tissue, has an 80% cure rate. Compared with other cancers, deaths from testicular cancer are rare. Treatment for testicular cancer includes the surgical removal of the affected testicle (which should not affect fertility or the ability to have sexual intercourse), chemotherapy and radiotherapy.

PUZZLE GRID

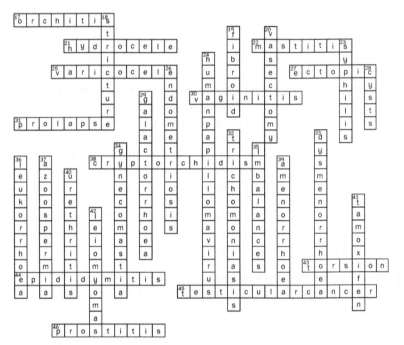

10 The integumentary system

INTRODUCTION

The skin is a complex organ consisting of three distinct layers (epidermis, dermis and subcutaneous) and accessory structures, such as hair and nails. When intact, the skin provides the body's first line of defence with respect to infection, as well as controlling body temperature and preventing excessive fluid loss.

Due to the prominence of the skin, its integrity is under constant threat. Skin disorders can be due to many factors, including trauma, allergy, infection, tumour and environmental stresses. They may also be degenerative, congenital or secondary to another illness or disease within another organ system. For example, acne can be attributed to a hormonal imbalance in the endocrine system but appears as lesions on the skin. Diagnosis of skin disorders sometimes involves taking a sample of affected tissue or collecting fluid from a lesion, and sensitivity patch testing on the skin is commonly used in allergy investigations.

In addition, the skin affords an important administrative route for a number of drugs, thus promoting both local and systemic effects.

The visibility of the skin, hair and nails makes them useful when assessing many conditions, and the characteristics of skin lesions are helpful when making a diagnosis. Furthermore, many nursing interventions involve the skin, so nurses should know and understand how the skin protects the body and assists in the maintenance of homoeostasis.

Useful resources

Nurses! Test Yourself in Anatomy and Physiology (2nd edition)
Chapter 3

Symptoms, Diagnosis and Treatment
Chapter 7

Gould's Pathophysiology for the Healthcare Professions (7th edition)
Chapter 8

LABELLING EXERCISE

1–5   Identify the type of skin lesions in Figure 10.1, using the terms in the box below:

---

vesicle   papule

ulcer   weal

pustule

Figure 10.1 Skin lesions

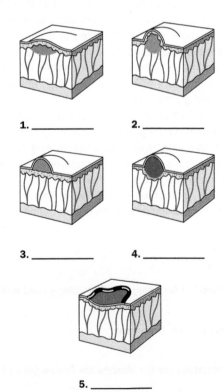

1. _____   2. _____

3. _____   4. _____

5. _____

TRUE OR FALSE?

Are the following statements true or false?

| 6 | A burrow is the primary lesion of varicella zoster. |

| 7 | There are three basic types of skin cancer. |

| 8 | Severe neuralgia is a frequent complication of the herpes simplex infection. |

| 9 | Laser therapy can be used in the treatment of warts. |

| 10 | Impetigo is an autoimmune condition. |

| 11 | A partial-thickness burn affects only the epidermis. |

| 12 | Infection by the varicella zoster virus leads to chickenpox. |

| 13 | Papular urticaria may be life-threatening. |

| 14 | Scabies is caused by a parasitic infection. |

| 15 | Infection occurs more frequently in closed wounds. |

MULTIPLE CHOICE

Identify one correct answer for each of the following:

16 Treatment of chronic urticaria includes the application of:
a) corticosteroids
b) antihistamines
c) menthol cream
d) all of these

17 An open wound is an injury that causes a break in which skin layer?
a) all skin layers
b) epidermis
c) dermis
d) subcutaneous

18 Which application is best for treating acute oozing skin conditions?
a) drying lotions
b) powders
c) ointments
d) creams

19 Moles may be considered sinister if:
a) they increase in size
b) they change in shape
c) they bleed
d) any of these occur

20 An emollient is:

    a) an antibiotic

    b) a steroid

    c) an alcohol-based medication

    d) a substance that moisturizes and soothes skin

21 Androgenetic alopecia can be treated with:

    a) oestrogens

    b) benzyl penicillin

    c) topical minoxidil

    d) spironolactone

22 The stages of deep wound healing occur in which order?

    a) migration, inflammation, proliferation, maturation

    b) inflammation, proliferation, migration, maturation

    c) inflammation, proliferation, maturation, migration

    d) inflammation, migration, proliferation, maturation

23 Which of the following is *not* part of the primary treatment for full-thickness burns?

    a) maintaining cosmetic appearance of skin

    b) replacing lost fluids and electrolytes

    c) providing dietary nutrients

    d) preventing infection

24 Onychomycosis refers to:

    a) ringworm of the scalp

    b) inflammation of sebaceous glands

    c) a fungal infection of the nail bed

    d) an area of necrotic tissue

25 Which of the following is *not* a risk factor for malignant melanoma ?

a) exposure to sunlight

b) dark skin

c) history of sunburn

d) family history

26 What abnormal skin colour might indicate rising levels of bilirubin?

a) yellow

b) blue

c) red

d) general paleness

MATCH THE TERMS

Classify each immune disorder listed below:

A. bacterial infection   **C.** fungal infection

B. viral infection   **D.** inflammation

---

27 Shingles _____

28 Eczema _____

29 Oral thrush _____

30 Impetigo _____

31 Cellulitis _____

32 Athlete's foot _____

33 Psoriasis _____

PUZZLE GRID

Use the word bank (below) and clues (overleaf) to solve the puzzle.

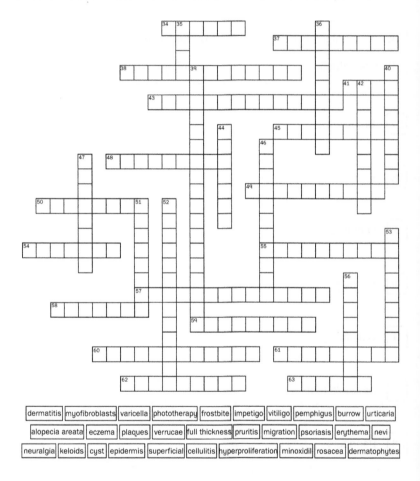

dermatitis | myofibroblasts | varicella | phototherapy | frostbite | impetigo | vitiligo | pemphigus | burrow | urticaria

alopecia areata | eczema | plaques | verrucae | full thickness | pruritis | migration | psoriasis | erythema | nevi

neuralgia | keloids | cyst | epidermis | superficial | cellulitis | hyperproliferation | minoxidil | rosacea | dermatophytes

Clues across

34 Group of conditions that cause the skin to become itchy, inflamed or have a rash-like appearance (6)

37 Acute infectious disease caused by a DNA virus that is a member of the herpesvirus group; chickenpox (9)

38 Type of burns trauma in which the epidermal and dermal layers of the skin are destroyed, and damage may even penetrate subcutaneous fat (4, 9)

41 Visible, circumscribed, chronic lesion of the skin or mucosa that may be either congenital or acquired (4)

43 Autoimmune disorder that usually results in unpredictable, patchy hair loss (8, 6)

45 Antihypertensive drug that may be used as a foam or topical solution to treat androgenetic hair loss (9)

48 Condition that occurs when a trigger causes high levels of histamine and other chemical messengers to be released in the skin (9)

49 Term used to describe several types of skin irritation and rashes caused by genetic influences, an overactive immune system, infections, allergies or irritating substances (10)

50 Hyperkeratotic lesions found esapecially over the pressure areas of the feet (8)

54 Raised scars that can occur where the skin has healed after an injury (7)

55 Common bacterial infection of the skin and underlying soft tissues that may occur following damage to the integrity of the skin (10)

Clues down

35 Closed capsule or sac-like structure within the skin, usually filled with liquid, semi-solid material (4)

36 Early event involving keratinocytes that is essential for wound re-epithelialization (9)

39 Abnormal growth of keratinocytes in psoriasis, resulting in the epidermal hyperplasia that is characteristic of psoriasis (18)

40 Condition in which the skin loses its melanocyte function, causing the appearance of pale white patches (8)

42 External zone of the skin that is the origin of both melanoma and non-melanoma cancers (9)

44 Raised, inflamed and scaly patches of skin that may also be itchy and painful that occur with some forms of psoriasis (7)

46 Type of burn in which trauma damage is limited to the epidermis (11)

47 Chronic itch associated with several disorders, including dry skin, infection, pregnancy and cancer (though rarely) (8)

51 Redness of the skin caused by injury or another inflammation-causing condition such as infection, abrasion or overexposure to the sun (8)

52 Fungi responsible for superficial infections of the skin, hair and nails (13)

53 Chronic skin disease that causes red, itchy scaly patches, most commonly on the knees, elbows, trunk and scalp (9)

Clues across (continued)

57 Main producers and organizers of the extracellular matrix essential for the restoration of tissue integrity after injury (14)

58 Chronic inflammatory skin condition that usually affects the face (7)

59 Severe facial pain due to an irritated or damaged nerve (9)

60 Medical treatment in which natural or artificial light is used to improve dermatological conditions such as psoriasis, eczema, dermatitis and vitiligo (12)

61 Rare group of autoimmune diseases that cause painful blisters to develop on the skin and lining of the mucous membranes (9)

62 Trauma to the skin that occurs when it is exposed to extreme low temperatures, causing freezing of peripheral tissues (9)

63 Irregular tracks in the web spaces between the fingers, on the palms and wrists caused by infestation with the parasitic mite, *Sarcoptes scabiei* (6)

Clues down (continued)

56 Common skin infection in children caused by *Staphylococcus aureus* or group A streptococcal bacteria (8)

ANSWERS

 LABELLING EXERCISE

Figure 10.2 Skin lesions

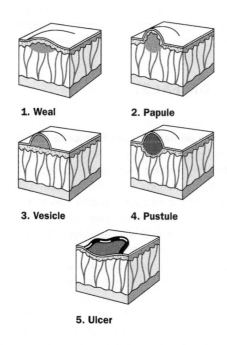

1. Weal

2. Papule

3. Vesicle

4. Pustule

5. Ulcer

[1] ***Weal (wheal):*** a localized elevation of the epidermis caused by an accumulation of fluid in the papillary dermis. An example of a weal lesion is urticaria (hives).

[2] ***Papule:*** a solid elevation of both the dermis and epidermal layers that contains fluid. An insect bite may cause a papule to develop. Nodules are large papules that sometimes extend into the subcutaneous layer, for example, a cyst.

3   *Vesicle (blister):* a papule located directly under the skin surface
that has filled with fluid. A large vesicle is sometimes called a bulla
(pl. bullae). Partial thickness (second degree) burns often form
vesicles.

4   *Pustule:* a lesion similar in size to a papule but filled with pus that
contains necrotic inflammatory cells. An acne blemish is an example
of a pustule.

5   *Ulcer (erosion):* can occur after a vesicle or pustule ruptures. Ulcers
have lost at least part of the epidermis. Examples include pressure
(bed) sores (also known as decubitus ulcers).

TRUE OR FALSE?

6   **A burrow is the primary lesion of varicella zoster.**   **X**
The primary lesions associated with varicella zoster infection are
small blister-like vesicles that are a characteristic of chickenpox.
A person with chickenpox is infectious from 1–5 days before the
rash appears. The contagious period continues until all the blisters have formed scabs, which may take 5–10 days. It takes from
10–21 days after contact with an infected person for someone to
develop chickenpox. In adults, chickenpox is often associated with
loss of appetite (anorexia), myalgia, nausea, fever, headache, sore
throat, earache, feeling pressure in the head, a swollen face and
malaise. In children, the first symptom is usually the appearance
of a papular rash, followed by development of malaise, fever and
loss of appetite. Less common symptoms include cough, rhinitis,
abdominal pain and gastrointestinal distress. Typically, the disease is more severe in adults. Burrows are a sign of infestation by
scabies-causing parasites.

7   **There are three basic types of skin cancer.**   **✔**
Skin cancers account for about 40% of all cancers. In recent years,
there has been a significant increase in the number of reported
cases. Basal cell carcinoma and squamous cell carcinoma are the
two most common types of skin cancer. The third type, malignant
melanoma, is a less frequent but more serious form of skin cancer
accountable for 4% of all skin cancer cases but around 80% of all

skin cancer deaths. Exposure to ultraviolet (UV) radiation causes most skin cancers by triggering genetic mutations. Areas of skin with wide exposure to the sun are at significant risk of skin cancer but protection from the sun significantly reduces risk. As with other cancers, skin cancer lesions progress through the stages of initiation, promotion, progression and metastasis.

8 | **Severe neuralgia is a frequent complication of the herpes simplex infection.**

Although neuralgia can occur after infection with the herpes simplex virus (HSV), it is generally mild and gives little cause for concern. However, other neurological syndromes have been linked to HSV infection, including epilepsy, multiple sclerosis, atypical pain syndromes, and ascending or transverse myelitis (inflammation of the spinal column). These are typically more serious.

9 | **Laser therapy can be used in the treatment of warts.**

Warts are benign lesions of the skin caused by the human papillomavirus (HPV), which most commonly occurs in children and young adults. The infection is acquired when the virus is introduced into the skin through defects in the epidermis. New treatments for warts involve using a pulsed dye laser, which selectively destroys warts without damaging the surrounding skin. The laser selectively destroys blood vessels that supply the wart, as well as thermally destroying the wart. Traditional treatments for warts involve physical destruction of the virally infected cell. These treatments include the application of acids (such as salicylic acid), liquid nitrogen therapy (cryosurgery), electrocautery and carbon dioxide ablation. These treatments all cause destruction of the top layer of the skin and may result in permanent scarring. In many cases, warts may be resistant to these kinds of therapy. Compared with alternative treatments, pulsed dye laser therapy is very safe and effective, even in warts that have become resistant to previous treatment.

10 | **Impetigo is an autoimmune condition.**

Impetigo is a highly contagious bacterial skin infection of the superficial layers of the skin. About 70% of infections occur in children, making it the most common childhood skin infection in the UK. It is caused by the *Staphylococcus aureus* or more rarely *Streptococcus pyogenes* bacteria. The first sign of impetigo is a patch of red, itchy skin. The condition is characterized by red sores, generally around the mouth and nose. The sores soon burst and ooze fluid or pus, forming a yellowish-brown crust, which leaves a red mark as it dries. The condition usually heals without scarring. Although the sores are not painful, they may be very itchy. To prevent the spread of infection (to other body parts or other people), it is important not to touch or scratch the affected area. Treatment is usually with topical or oral antibiotics and good hygiene. In rare cases, symptoms may be more severe, and the patient may develop a fever and swollen glands.

11 | **A partial-thickness burn affects only the epidermis.** ✗

In recent years, classification of burns by burn depth has changed. Injury to the epidermis (top or outer skin layer) is now called a superficial burn (formerly called a first-degree burn). Injury to the dermis (second layer) is now called a partial-thickness or dermal injury (formerly a second-degree burn). An injury that extends down to the third layer (the subcutaneous tissue, which includes fat) is called a full-thickness injury (formerly a third-degree burn). Burns that damage muscles underneath the subcutaneous skin layer are also described as full-thickness burns (formerly a fourth-degree burn). Full-thickness burns tend to be less painful than superficial and partial-thickness burns because the sensory nerves may have been damaged or destroyed by a full-thickness burn.

Superficial burns normally heal within 5–7 days. A common type of superficial burn is sunburn. Since the epidermis is thin (about the thickness of a piece of paper), it is easily replaced. Even when skin is not injured, the epidermis is completely replaced every 45–75 days. Healing from a superficial burn usually occurs without scarring, although there may be some permanent discoloration. The dermis is 15–40 times thicker than the epidermis, so the seriousness of a partial thickness (or dermal) burn depends on the depth to which the dermis has been injured. Partial-thickness burns usually leave scars. Deep and large partial-thickness burns will usually require skin grafting. A full-thickness burn destroys all three layers of skin, resulting in the loss of not only the skin but also the accessory structures such as hair follicles, sweat glands, and the region where new skin cells are formed. For these reasons, full-thickness burns require skin grafts. Full-thickness burns extend through the skin into underlying tissues, such as ligaments and muscle; these are often life-threatening.

12 **Infection by the varicella zoster virus leads to chickenpox.**
Chickenpox is a highly contagious illness caused by primary infection with the varicella zoster virus. It usually starts with a vesicle skin rash, mainly on the body and head rather than at the periphery, which develops into itchy raw lesions that mostly heal without scarring. Chickenpox is rarely fatal, although it is generally more severe in adult males than in adult females or children. Pregnant women and those with a suppressed immune system are at highest risk of serious complications. Chickenpox is now believed to be the cause of one-third of stroke cases in children. The most common future complication of chickenpox is shingles, caused by reactivation of the varicella zoster virus decades after the initial episode of chickenpox. Following primary infection, there is usually lifelong protective immunity from further episodes of chickenpox.

13 **Papular urticaria may be life-threatening.**
Urticaria is the clinical name for hives. Papules may open when scratched and become crusty and infected. Papular urticaria is a common disorder in children, manifested by chronic or recurrent papules caused by an allergic hypersensitivity reaction to insects (for example, mosquitoes). Treatment is usually with oral antihistamines and oral corticosteroids, such as prednisolone.

14 **Scabies is caused by a parasitic infection.**
Scabies is a contagious skin infection caused by tiny parasitic mites that burrow into the skin and lay eggs. Symptoms include intense itch (sometimes worse at night) and skin rash indicating where the mites have burrowed. Diagnosis is usually from observing the skin, although a skin sample may be taken and examined for the parasitic mites and their eggs. Insecticide creams are used to treat the parasitic infection, with permethrin cream usually recommended as the first treatment option; however, it should only be used under medical supervision if pregnant or breastfeeding and in children under 2 years. Malathion lotion is used if the permethrin cream is ineffective; it has no known effects during pregnancy and breastfeeding. Treating scabies also involves educating patients properly about correct hygiene to limit the spread of infection. Scabies tends to be more common where many people are in close proximity, such as schools and nursing homes.

15 **Infection occurs more frequently in closed wounds.**   **X**
Closed wounds can affect any internal tissue but the epithelium is intact and so infection is less likely to occur. A common example of a closed wound is a bruise (contusion) caused by bleeding in the dermis. A facial contusion may be relatively harmless or can indicate more serious internal injury such as intracranial bleeding. Closed wounds affecting organs or organ systems are often life-threatening.

MULTIPLE CHOICE
Correct answers identified in *bold italics*

16 **Treatment of chronic urticaria includes the application of:**
a) corticosteroids   b) antihistamines
c) menthol cream   ***d) all of these***

Urticaria is the clinical name for hives, which appear as an area of raised erythema and oedema of the superficial dermis and are frequently associated with type I hypersensitivity reactions. The lesions are mediated by release of histamine and may appear as weals, welts or hives. Chronic urticaria can be treated with antihistamines, corticosteroids, and menthol cream. Patients should also be advised to avoid triggers where possible.

17 **An open wound is an injury that causes a break in which skin layer?**
a) all skin layers   ***b) epidermis***
c) dermis   d) subcutaneous

An open wound is exposed to the external environment, meaning the outer epidermal layer has been broken. In a closed wound (such as a bruise), the epidermis remains intact. Several types of open wounds exist (Figure 10.3).

I. *Abrasion*: a superficial wound over a large area usually caused by scraping against a solid object. There may be only slight bleeding, leaving this type of wound open to infection.

II. *Avulsion*: a considerable amount of tissue is torn away with great force. It is usually associated with amputation injuries where considerable bleeding and serious internal damage may occur.

Figure 10.3 Common open wounds

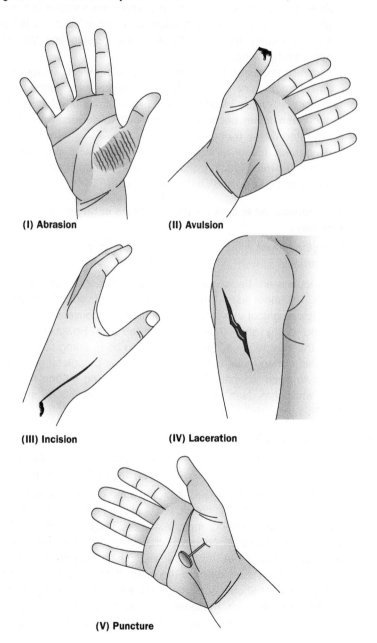

(I) Abrasion

(II) Avulsion

(III) Incision

(IV) Laceration

(V) Puncture

III. *Incision*: a linear cut by a sharp object (such as a knife wound). Bleeding can be severe if deep vessels are severed but such bleeding can help clean the wound and limit infection. It is usually stitched or bandaged to close the incision and limit the opportunity for infection.

IV. *Laceration*: caused by impact from a solid object. Tissue damage is more extensive because of the irregular, jagged tear. Despite extensive bleeding, there is a high risk of infection. Tissue often scars because it is difficult to correctly reposition lacerated tissue for healing.

V. *Puncture*: caused by slender, pointed objects, a puncture produces minimal bleeding, thus any invading pathogens can easily enter the body and cause infection.

18 **Which application is best for treating acute oozing skin conditions?**

a) ***drying lotions*** b) powders
c) ointments d) creams

Drying lotions are usually applied to acute oozing or weeping skin lesions. The most used lotions contain alcohol, propylene glycol, polyethylene glycol or water. These lotions are convenient to apply and tend to dry rather than moisturize the skin. However, depending on the vehicle used, these lotions can be irritating to the skin, particularly when those containing alcohol and propylene glycol are applied to open wounds. The opposite of drying lotions is emollients, which are used to moisturize dry skin conditions such as dermatitis (eczema) or psoriasis.

19 **Moles are considered sinister if:**

a) they increase in size b) they change in shape
c) they bleed d) ***any of these occur***

Moles (or nevi) are defined as a proliferation of melanocytes. Normally they are brownish in colour, flat or slightly raised, have smooth borders, and have a uniform pigmentation. They are normally less than 6 mm in diameter. Abnormal characteristics of moles include asymmetry, changes in the border and colour, increased diameter and elevation, or bleeding from the mole. If any of these changes develop, patients should seek medical advice, since it may indicate a malignant melanoma. Malignant melanomas are the most prevalent life-threatening cancer in middle-aged adults. These cancers metastasize rapidly and have an extremely poor prognosis. Early recognition of cutaneous melanomas can have a major positive impact on surgical cure.

20 An emollient is:

a) an antibiotic
b) a steroid
c) an alcohol-based medication
d) a substance that moisturizes and soothes skin

An emollient is an agent that soothes and softens the skin, such as lanolin or liquid paraffin. Emollients are used alone as moisturizers to reduce the need for active drug therapy (such as corticosteroids for eczema) and in skin preparations as a base for more active drugs, such as antibiotics.

21 Androgenetic alopecia can be treated with:

a) oestrogens   b) benzyl penicillin
c) topical minoxidil   d) spironolactone

Androgenetic (or androgenic) alopecia is a degenerative skin disorder that affects both males and females. Minoxidil is a vasodilator medication that slows or stops hair loss and promotes hair regrowth. It is available over the counter for treatment of androgenetic alopecia, among other hair loss treatments, but measurable changes disappear within months after discontinuation of treatment. The mechanism by which minoxidil promotes hair growth is not fully understood. Minoxidil is also a vasodilator. It is speculated that by widening blood vessels and opening potassium channels, it allows more blood, and therefore oxygen and nutrients, to enter the follicle. It is less effective when there is a large area of hair loss. In addition, its effectiveness has largely been demonstrated in younger men (aged 18–41 years). Minoxidil use is indicated for central (vertex) hair loss only.

22 The stages in deep wound healing occur in which order?

a) migration, inflammation, proliferation, maturation
b) inflammation, proliferation, migration, maturation
c) inflammation, proliferation, maturation, migration
d) inflammation, migration, proliferation, maturation

Deep wound healing involves several phases and is more complex than primary or epidermal healing, which is repaired by enlargement and migration of basal cells, contact inhibition, and division of migrating and stationary basal cells. In deep wound healing, the initial phase involves inflammation, a vascular and cellular response that prepares tissue for repair. During the inflammatory phase, a blood clot forms in the wound, uniting the damaged tissue edges. Vasodilation and increased permeability of blood vessels enhance the delivery of white cells that remove microbes and debris and mesenchymal cells which develop into fibroblasts.

In the subsequent migration phase, the clot develops into a scab and epithelial cells migrate beneath the scab to bridge the wound. Newly formed fibroblasts migrate along fibrin threads and begin producing scar tissue containing collagen and glycoproteins. Damaged blood vessels also begin to grow at this stage. The proliferation phase is characterized by an extensive growth of epithelial cells beneath the scab, further deposition of collagen fibres and continued blood vessel growth. The final maturation phase involves the sloughing of the scab once the epidermis is restored to normal thickness. Collagen fibres become more organized in their pattern of deposition and fibroblasts decrease in number.

Scar tissue formation is called fibrosis. Depending on the extent of the wound, excess scar tissue may be formed resulting in raised scar formation, which may remain within the boundaries of the original wound (hypertrophic scar) or it may extend into surrounding normal tissues (keloid scar). Scar tissue differs from normal skin since it frequently has fewer blood vessels and contains no hair, glandular tissue or sensory neurones.

23 | **Which of the following is *not* part of the primary treatment for full-thickness burns?**

a) *maintaining cosmetic appearance of skin*
b) replacing lost fluids and electrolytes
c) providing dietary nutrients
d) preventing infection

Most full-thickness burns cause severe damage to the skin and so often require skin grafts at a later stage because the skin cannot replace itself. Lots of fluids are lost by burns patients, so replacing fluids and electrolytes is very important in their treatment. Fluids are also important for thermoregulation to maintain an optimum body temperature. Nutrition is very important to provide the correct nutrients and energy for healing and also for thermoregulation.

Infection control is essential because the broken skin provides an opportunity for invading pathogens to enter the body. Widespread infection can cause septicaemia, which is the main cause of death in burns patients.

24 **Onychomycosis refers to:**

a) ringworm of the scalp
b) inflammation of sebaceous glands
c) *a fungal infection of the nail bed*
d) an area of necrotic tissue

Onychomycosis (fungal nail infection) is the most common disease of the nails and contributes to about a half of all nail abnormalities. It may affect toenails or fingernails, but toenail infections are most common. Symptoms include a thickened, yellow or cloudy nail-plate. The nails can become rough and crumbly or can separate from the nail bed. There is usually no pain or other symptoms, unless the disease is severe but patients with onychomycosis may experience significant psychosocial problems due to the appearance of the nail, particularly when fingernails are affected.

The pathogen that commonly causes onychomycosis is the yeast *Candida*, which enters a damaged or cracked nail. It is more common in older people. Treating onychomycosis is challenging because the infection is embedded within the nail and is difficult to reach. As a result, full eradication of symptoms is very slow and may take a year or more. Most treatments are either systemic antifungal medications such as terbinafine and itraconazole, or a topical such as nail paints containing salicylic acid, tioconazole or amorolfine. There is also evidence for combining systemic and topical treatments. Newer therapies include treatment with laser light sources, which kill the fungus in the nail bed.

25 **Which of the following is not a risk factor for malignant melanoma?**

a) exposure to sunlight   *b)* *dark skin*
c) history of sunburn   d) family history

Melanoma is a malignant tumour of the skin that is increasing in frequency. Risk factors for the disease include a genetic predisposition, exposure to UV light (from sun or artificial sunbeds), steroid hormone activity, a fair complexion that burns easily in the sun and freckles. Wearing a sun lotion with a high sun protection factor

(SPF) will help reduce skin damage from UV light. Melanomas arise because of malignant degeneration of melanocytes located in the basal layer of the epidermis.

26 **What abnormal skin colour might indicate rising levels of bilirubin?**

a) yellow   b) blue   c) red   d) general paleness

A yellow colouring in skin indicates the presence of jaundice, resulting from increased bilirubin levels in blood. Except for physiological jaundice in the newborn, this condition does not normally occur. The condition in the child or adult may be first noted in the junction of the hard and soft palate in the mouth and in the sclera (whites) of the eyes. As levels of serum bilirubin rise, jaundice becomes more evident over the rest of the body.

Other skin colours indicate a range of abnormal physiological states:

- Erythema, an intense redness of the skin, is often associated with inflammation or fever and is related to an increased rate of blood flow through the surface vessels.
- Cyanosis is characterized by a bluish colour and often signifies decreased tissue perfusion that may be due to anaemia or inadequate blood flow.
- General paleness (pallor) may indicate acute anxiety or fear, and results from the peripheral vasoconstriction that occurs with sympathetic nervous system stimulation. Skin can also appear pale due to vasoconstriction from exposure to cold or pallor may be caused by oedema.

MATCH THE TERMS

27 Shingles   **B. viral infection**

- *Pathophysiology*: Shingles (herpes zoster) describes an infection of a nerve and its surrounding tissue. Shingles is characterized by a skin rash of tiny but painful fluid-filled blisters. It can affect any part of the body, including the face.
- *Risk factors*: Patients must previously have been infected with the varicella zoster virus (usually during an episode of chickenpox). The virus remains dormant in the body after the illness but can be reactivated later in life. Reactivation of the virus is

thought to be associated with reduced immunity; therefore, immuno-compromised patients are at risk. Stress is also a risk factor.

- *Causes*: It is caused by the varicella zoster virus that also causes chickenpox, although it is not triggered by exposure to the virus. After having chickenpox, the virus remains dormant in the body but can be reactivated later, causing shingles. Unlike chickenpox, shingles is not contagious. However, if someone who has never had chickenpox is in contact with shingles, they can catch the virus from the shingles patient and develop chickenpox.

- *Symptoms*: The initial symptoms include pain and paraesthesia (pins and needles), followed by red rash that develops on the face, neck, shoulders and back (similar to the chickenpox rash). The scabs that form over the blisters can scar if scratched. The rash usually takes 2–4 weeks to disappear. These symptoms can be accompanied by exhaustion. Local symptoms are alleviated with cool compresses or calamine lotion. Persistent pain may be a debilitating complication of this condition, particularly in the older adult.

- *Diagnosis and treatment*: Diagnosis is usually from symptoms and there is not usually any formal testing. However, if the condition affects the eyes, a patient may be referred. Treatment is aimed at easing symptoms. Rash and scabs should be kept clean and dry. Patients should wear loose clothing to reduce itching, which can be treated topically with calamine lotion or orally with antihistamines. Paracetamol or ibuprofen can be used to treat mild-to-moderate pain, with opioids (such as codeine) being prescribed for more severe pain. Antiviral medications such as acyclovir help reduce the severity of the illness by stopping the virus from spreading; however, they are most effective if taken within 3 days of the rash appearing.

- *Complications*: There is risk of the blisters becoming infected, particularly if scratched a lot. Other complications include encephalitis (inflammation of the brain), transverse myelitis (inflammation of the spinal cord) or severe persistent nerve pain (neuralgia).

| 28 | Eczema | **D. inflammation** |

- *Pathophysiology*: Eczema is a form of the inflammatory skin condition dermatitis that causes inflammation of the papillary layer. There are several different types but the most common is atopic eczema, which mainly affects children and is associated with hypersensitivity reactions.

- *Risk factors*: Atopic eczema tends to be inherited and is associated with allergies, although it tends to disappear as the child gets older.
- *Causes*: As with all forms of dermatitis, the causes and triggers vary between patients. Common triggers include detergents, pet hair and certain foods such as dairy products.
- *Symptoms*: Dry, flaky skin that is sometimes itchy. During a flare-up, symptoms worsen, the skin can become hot (due to the inflammatory reaction) and may ooze or weep, which can become infected.
- *Diagnosis and treatment:* There are no formal diagnostic tests; diagnosis is usually made by examining the symptoms and taking a thorough history of known allergens and any similar family history. Treatment is usually aimed at preventing flare-ups by avoiding known triggers. Emollient creams can be prescribed to moisten skin. During a flare-up, a corticosteroid may be prescribed to reduce inflammation and an antibiotic may be required for any infection.

29   Oral thrush   **C. fungal infection**

- *Pathophysiology*: Oral thrush (candidiasis) is a fungal infection describing the presence of the *Candida* fungus in the mucous membranes of the mouth.
- *Risk factors*: It occurs more often in infants than adults, although it is unusual for breast-fed infants to develop oral thrush. For bottle-fed babies, all teats should be replaced to reduce recurrence of infection. In adults and older children, it is less common, although it can be common in denture-wearers. Mouth care is particularly important in chemotherapy patients and patients who receive radiotherapy to the head and neck. Certain antibiotics and other medications (such as steroids for asthma) can also be a risk factor.
- *Symptoms*: Formation of creamy white spots (plaques) in the mouth that when scraped off, reveal shallow ulcers. The underlying mucous membrane is red and tender and may bleed when plaques are removed. The tongue may also have a dense white coating. Babies may drool saliva or refuse to eat, while adults may experience soreness or a burning sensation in the mouth.

- *Diagnosis and treatment*: Oral thrush is usually diagnosed by simply looking in the mouth. It generally responds quickly to antifungal treatments such as miconazole gel, drops or pastilles. In adults and older children, predisposing causes should be investigated and treated first to prevent recurrence.

| 30 | Impetigo | **A. bacterial infection** |

- *Pathophysiology*: Impetigo is a superficial lesion of the skin usually caused by the bacteria Staphlococcus aureus or Streptococcus pyrogenes. There are two types of impetigo: non-bullous and bullous lesions. Non-bullous lesions account for about 70% of cases and are characterized by sores that rupture, leaving a yellow-brown crust. Bullous impetigo exhibits large fluid-filled blisters that are painless.
- *Risk factors*: It is most common in pre-school children and highly contagious. It is also common in patients with skin conditions such as scabies, nappy rash, dermatitis or eczema.
- *Causes*: Most cases are caused by Staphylococcus aureus, which invades the skin through an open wound such as a cut or bite. Bacteria penetrate the skin and cause an infection. When the blisters produce fluid, this indicates they are still infectious.
- *Symptoms*: Lesions commonly occur on the face and begin as small vesicles that rapidly enlarge and rupture to form yellow-brown crusts. Underneath this characteristic crust, the lesion is red and moist and may exude fluid. Additional vesicles develop around the primary site and itching is common.
- *Diagnosis and treatment*: Diagnosis is usually by observing symptoms and excluding other skin conditions such as cellulitis, scabies and chickenpox. If the infection does not respond to treatment, a sample may be taken to exclude other conditions. Topical antibiotics may be used on clean, dry skin using gloves to prevent spread of infection. Oral antibiotics may be prescribed for a severe or rapidly spreading infection. With treatment, the infection usually clears within a week. Since it is contagious, infected children should be kept out of school/nursery; towels should not be shared and should be laundered after each use until the infection has cleared.
- *Complications*: Although rare, cellulitis can develop, which can lead to septicaemia.

31 Cellulitis **A. bacterial infection**

- *Pathophysiology*: Cellulitis is an infection of the dermis and subcutaneous tissues usually caused by staphlococci or streptococci.
- *Causes and risk factors*: A skin wound such as an ulcer, boil (furuncle) or carbuncle (abscess larger than a boil) can allow bacteria to enter the deeper tissues, causing infection and inflammation. Risk factors include diabetes mellitus, oedema and peripheral vascular disease.
- *Symptoms*: Hot, red, swollen and painful area, with itching, burning and tenderness as the infection develops. This may be accompanied by fever and chills as the bacteria release their toxins. There may be a clear line observed where the cellulitis stops but spreading of this line can be observed as the infection spreads. Oozing and pus at the wound site can occur but this is less common.
- *Diagnosis and treatment*: Diagnosis is usually made by assessing the symptoms. If there is an open wound, a sample may be taken to identify the bacteria. Systemic antibiotics are required to treat the infection, which can become severe and even life-threatening if left untreated.
- *Complications*: Certain individuals are more susceptible to cellulitis such as diabetics and immuno-compromised patients. If the infection enters the blood, the patient is at risk of septicaemia (blood poisoning), which can be fatal if not treated urgently.

32 Athlete's foot **C. fungal infection**

- *Pathophysiology*: Athlete's foot (tinea pedis) is a mild superficial fungal infection of the foot and is quite common in adults. It causes a rash to develop, particularly between the toes but it can spread to the nails.
- *Causes*: It is caused by fungi that grow in warm, moist conditions.
- *Risk factors*: Athlete's foot is highly contagious and is associated with showers and swimming pools.
- *Symptoms*: An itchy, flaky rash between the toes that can smell. Deep cracks (fissures) can develop in the skin extending from the epidermis into the dermis, exposing new tissue, which can be painful and increase the risk of bacterial infection. Symptoms usually disappear in 10 days when treated.
- *Diagnosis and treatment*: Mild infection is usually diagnosed by observing of the skin of the foot (sometimes with a UV light).

Mild infections can be treated with over-the-counter antifungal (miconazole or clotrimazole) powders and creams. For more severe symptoms, a sample may be taken, and treatment may include both topical and systemic antifungal medication. A severe rash may also need a hydrocortisone cream.

- *Complications*: Infection can spread to the toenail, which can become infected with bacteria. This can lead to cellulitis.

33 Psoriasis   D. Inflammation

- *Pathophysiology*: Psoriasis is a chronic inflammatory skin disorder that is a form of hyperkeratosis, which is characterized by excessive production of keratin when skin cells replace themselves too quickly. The life cycle to grow and replace normal skin cells is approximately 28 days. In psoriasis, this cycle is accelerated, occurring as rapidly as every 2–6 days, meaning dead cells accumulate on the skin surface, producing the characteristic scaly patches. There are several different types of psoriasis, of which plaque psoriasis accounts for the majority of cases.
- *Risk factors*: Plaque psoriasis is not contagious, although there is a strong genetic link. Patients tend to become familiar with the triggers that cause their condition to flare up. Triggers include stress, smoking, alcohol, certain medicines (such as ibuprofen) and in response to skin injuries such as sunburn.
- *Causes*: The causes of psoriasis are not well known, although there is evidence to suggest it is due to an autoimmune response that attacks healthy skin cells and speeds up the cycle of cell replication.
- *Symptoms*: Red, flaky crusty patches of skin covered in silver scales. Patches are usually quite small and can appear anywhere on the body, although they are more common on the knees, elbows and scalp. Psoriasis can itch but it is not usually severe.
- *Diagnosis and treatment*: Diagnosis is usually by symptoms and determining if there is a family history. In rare cases, a skin sample may be taken to determine the type of psoriasis and to exclude other possible conditions. There is no cure for psoriasis, so treatment is aimed at easing symptoms using topical emollient creams to moisturize skin. In more severe cases, phototherapy using UV light can help reduce symptoms but this should be conducted under medical supervision.

PUZZLE GRID

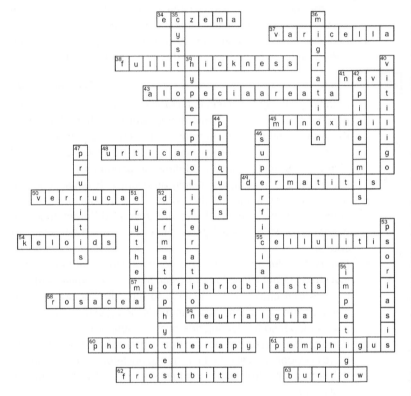

11 The musculoskeletal system

INTRODUCTION

The musculoskeletal system provides structure and support to the body, allowing it to move. It consists of bones, muscle, joints, cartilage, tendons and ligaments. There are three major types of muscle: smooth, skeletal and cardiac muscle. However, only skeletal muscle is involved with movement of the skeleton. There are five types of bone, classified by shape and location, which perform physiological and mechanical functions.

Some diseases and disorders of the musculoskeletal system have a very gradual onset, such as the autoimmune disorder rheumatoid arthritis, while others can be acute, such as fractures. With a gradual onset, patients may have no apparent symptoms for many years, yet damage may be occurring. Most diseases or disorders of this system are diagnosed through X-ray or other bone scans such as computerized tomography (CT), magnetic resonance imaging (MRI) or bone density scanning. With fractures, it is important not to exacerbate the break; ideally, patients should not be moved until the limb is splinted.

Many musculoskeletal conditions are chronic, and treatment involves controlling symptoms and slowing progression. In fractures, it is important to align and immobilize the broken bone quickly so that healing can begin.

Nurses should appreciate the essential role of the musculoskeletal system in controlling the internal and external movements of the body. It is important to remember that the anatomy and physiology of the musculoskeletal system are influenced by other systems and that disorders of these can affect the body's muscles and skeleton.

Useful resources

Nurses! Test Yourself in Anatomy and Physiology (2nd edition)
Chapter 11

Ross and Wilson's Anatomy and Physiology in Health and Illness (14th edition)
Chapter 16

LABELLING EXERCISE

1–9 Identify the different kinds of fractures in Figure 11.1, using the terms provided in the box below.

buckle	impacted	comminuted
crush	pathological	spiral
greenstick	compound	simple

Figure 11.1 Fracture types

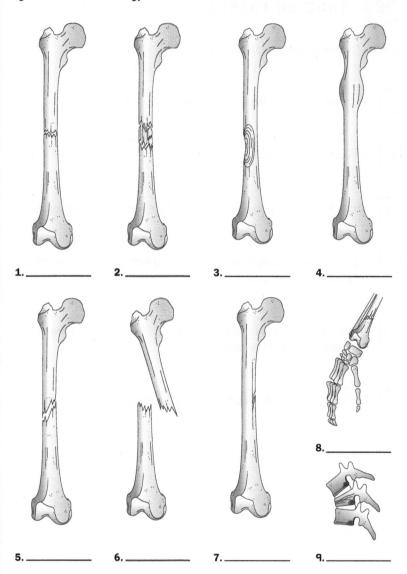

1. _____

2. _____

3. _____

4. _____

5. _____

6. _____

7. _____

8. _____

9. _____

TRUE OR FALSE?

Are the following statements true or false?

10 Tenosynovitis describes inflammation of a tendon.

11 A longitudinal fracture is a break across the diameter of the bone.

12 Strain is the injury caused to a bone by overexertion or overuse.

13 A person with a suspected fracture may look pale and clammy and feel faint, dizzy or sick.

14 Osteoporosis is a metabolic disease of the skeleton characterized by a reduction in bone density.

15 Osteoarthritis can be cured with nonsteroidal anti-inflammatory drugs.

16 Osteoarthritis is triggered by acute inflammation.

MULTIPLE CHOICE

Identify one correct answer for each of the following:

17 What type of fracture describes a bone that does not break completely?

a) stress fracture

b) compression fracture

c) fracture dislocation

d) hairline fracture

18 Each of the following represents a type of inflammatory arthritis, with the exception of:

a) rheumatoid arthritis

b) osteoarthritis

c) lupus

d) osteomyelitis

19 Which of the following tests is most commonly used to confirm a fracture?

a) bone density scan

b) MRI scan

c) CT scan

d) X-ray

20 Which of the following tests is used to diagnose osteoporosis?

a) bone density scan

b) CT scan

c) X-ray

d) MRI scan

21 Which of the following is often the first specific symptom of osteoporosis?

a) unexplained fracture

b) joint pain

c) limb stiffness

d) nerve pain

22 Osteoporosis usually affects who?

a) pregnant women

b) older males

c) children

d) post-menopausal females

23 Which of the following does *not* contribute to carpal tunnel syndrome?

a) heart failure

b) renal failure

c) rheumatoid arthritis

d) diabetes mellitus

24 Which of the following drugs are used in treating carpal tunnel syndrome?

a) morphine

b) nonsteroidal anti-inflammatory

c) aspirin

d) paracetamol

25 Which of the following is *not* considered an initial symptom of osteoarthritis?

a) limited movement in affected joints

b) pain

c) joint stiffness after wakening

d) muscle-wasting

26 An inability to relax muscle following contraction is a feature of which type of muscular dystrophy?

a) Duchenne

b) myotonic

c) congenital

d) limb-girdle

FILL IN THE BLANKS

Fill in the blanks in each statement using the options in this box.
Not all of them are required, so choose carefully!

calcium	carpal tunnel syndrome	X-rayed
multiple sclerosis	hernia	aligned
genetic	magnesium	muscular dystrophy

27 The most common form of nerve entrapment conditions is _____ _____ _____.

28 A _____ occurs when an internal part of the body, such as an organ, pushes through a weakness in the muscle or surrounding tissue wall.

29 _____ _____ describes a group of inherited diseases characterized by progressive degeneration of groups of muscles.

30 Approximately 40–60% of patients with osteoarthritis will have a _____ link.

31 In addition to bisphosphonate drugs, a _____ supplement may be prescribed if bone density is low.

32 To treat fractures, the broken bones must first be _____; this is known as 'reducing' the fracture.

PUZZLE GRID

Use the word bank and clues (below) to solve the puzzle.

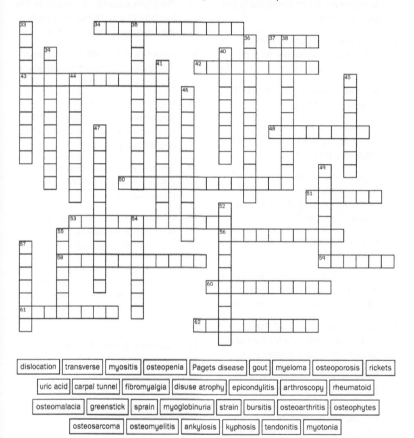

| dislocation | transverse | myositis | osteopenia | Pagets disease | gout | myeloma | osteoporosis | rickets |

| uric acid | carpal tunnel | fibromyalgia | disuse atrophy | epicondylitis | arthroscopy | rheumatoid |

| osteomalacia | greenstick | sprain | myoglobinuria | strain | bursitis | osteoarthritis | osteophytes |

| osteosarcoma | osteomyelitis | ankylosis | kyphosis | tendonitis | myotonia |

Clues across

34 Significant softening of the bones, most often caused by severe vitamin D deficiency (12)

Clues down

33 Trauma injury in which the ends of bones are forced from their normal positions (11)

Clues across (continued)

37 Form of arthritis that causes sudden, severe joint pain as a result of uric acid crystal formation in the joint space (4)

42 Inflammation or irritation of the thick fibrous cords that attach muscle to bone (10)

43 Most common type of cancer that originates in the bones (12)

48 Product of purine metabolism that may crystallize in the joints, causing gout (4, 4)

50 Common condition characterized by the gradual wearing down of cartilage, causing stiffness and pain in the joints (14)

51 Result of stretching or tearing of ligaments (6)

53 Inflammation or swelling that occurs in the bone often as a result of bacterial or fungal infection (13)

56 Descriptive of a type of fracture that occurs when the fracture line is perpendicular to the shaft (10)

58 Common syndrome characterized by pain, numbness and tingling in the hand and arm that occurs when the median nerve is compressed as it travels through the wrist (6, 6)

59 Injury that occurs through overstretched or torn muscles (6)

60 Autoimmune condition that affects the lining of the joints, causing a painful swelling that can result in bone erosion and joint deformity (10)

61 Group of rare conditions characterized by weak, painful or aching muscles (8)

Clues down (continued)

35 Pain that radiates from the elbow to the wrist on the medial side of the elbow caused by damage to the tendons that bend the wrist towards the palm; golfer's elbow (13)

36 Presence of myoglobin in the urine that may result from rhabdomyolysis or muscle injury (13)

38 Major cause of fractures in postmenopausal women caused by a reduction in bone mineral density and mass (12)

39 Surgical procedure used in the diagnosis and treatment of joint problems (11)

40 Condition in which condylar movement is restricted because of fusion of intra-articular joint components (9)

41 Chronic disease of the skeleton that affects bone remodelling, resulting in the formation of new bone that is abnormally shaped, weak and brittle (6, 7)

44 Low bone density than may eventually lead to osteoporosis (10)

45 Painful condition that affects the small, fluid-filled sacs that cushion the bones, tendons and muscles near joints (8)

46 Disorder characterized by widespread musculoskeletal pain accompanied by fatigue, sleep and memory issues, as well as depression (12)

47 Muscle wasting resulting in a decrease in muscle mass that may occur when a muscle is no longer as active as usual (6, 7)

49 Abnormal curvature of the spine (8)

Clues across (continued)

62 Fracture that occurs when a bone bends and cracks, rather than breaking completely into separate pieces (10)

Clues down (continued)

52 Lumps or spurs that grow on the bones of the spine or around joints affected by osteoarthritis (11)

54 Neuromuscular condition in which the relaxation of a muscle is impaired (8)

55 Softening and weakening of bones in children, usually a result of prolonged vitamin D deficiency (7)

57 Cancer that forms in blood plasma cells; Kahler's disease (7)

ANSWERS

 LABELLING EXERCISE

Figure 11.2 Fracture types

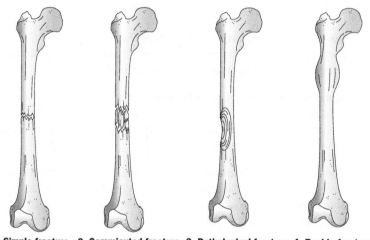

1. Simple fracture   2. Comminuted fracture   3. Pathological fracture   4. Buckle fracture

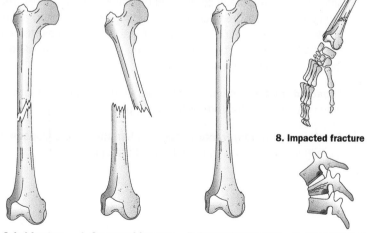

8. Impacted fracture

9. Crush fracture

5. Spiral fracture   6. Compound fracture   7. Greenstick fracture

1   **Simple (closed) fracture:** a clean break where the bone is broken in one place and does not damage surrounding tissue or penetrate the skin.

2   **Comminuted fracture:** the bone shatters into pieces. This type of splinter fracture is difficult to heal and occurs more commonly in serious accidents, such as a depressed fracture of the skull, where the fragment is pushed into the brain.

3   **Pathological fracture:** can occur in a bone weakened by a disease, such as osteoporosis, or by a tumour or cyst.

4   **Buckle (torus) fracture:** occurs commonly in children when the bone deforms but does not crack. It is painful but stable and tends to heal more quickly than greenstick factures.

5   **Spiral fracture:** caused by a twisting motion which results in a winding or slanting break. An oblique fracture (not pictured) is a diagonal fracture of the shaft along the bone's long axis, usually caused by a high impact.

6   **Compound (open) fracture:** occurs when the fractured bone pieces penetrate the skin, damaging surrounding soft tissue. Since the skin is broken there is a higher risk of infection, meaning this kind of fracture is more serious.

7   **Greenstick fracture:** occurs when the bone partly fractures on one side but does not break completely (an incomplete fracture). These are common in children because the young bone is softer, more elastic and able to bend. Greenstick fractures take longer to heal than buckle fractures because they tend to occur in the middle of the bone, which is slower growing.

8   **Impacted fracture:** fragments of bone are driven into each other (such as a Colles' fracture of the wrist, pictured).

9   **Crush (compression) fracture:** occurs when the bone collapses. It usually happens in the spongy bone of the spine.

TRUE OR FALSE?

10 **Tenosynovitis describes inflammation of a tendon.**

Tenosynovitis refers to the inflammation of the sheath that surrounds a tendon, rather than the tendon itself. Tendonitis is inflammation (swelling) of a tendon that causes pain in affected areas. It is more common in the tendons around the shoulder (supraspinatus tendonitis), elbow (tennis elbow), wrist, finger, thigh, knee or back of the heel (Achilles tendonitis). It is usually caused by overuse of the affected tendon, making it a common sports-related injury, although it can affect anyone. Older adults are also at risk of tendonitis because tendons lose elasticity and become weaker over time. Tendonitis and tenosynovitis can occur simultaneously.

11 **A longitudinal fracture is a break across the diameter of the bone.**

Longitudinal fractures occur along the length of the bone, while transverse fractures occur across the bone. An oblique fracture is a diagonal fracture of the shaft along the bone's long axis, usually caused by a high impact.

12 **Strain is the injury caused to a bone by overexertion or overuse.**

Strain is an injury caused to muscle fibres that stretch or tear due to overuse or overexertion, a common example being hamstring strain. Strains can be prevented by warming up before exercising. Sprains occur when one or more ligaments are stretched, twisted or torn, usually because of excessive force being applied to a joint. Sprains commonly occur at the knee, ankle and wrist. Mild and moderate strains and sprains are usually treated by following the PRICE procedure:

P = prevention by warming up
R = resting the muscle after injury
I = applying an ice pack in short bursts to reduce inflammation
C = compression with elastic strapping to reduce swelling and inflammation
E = keep the limb elevated to minimize pain and swelling.

Most people recover normal function 6–8 weeks after a sprain. However, the outlook for strains depends on the severity of the injury and in very severe cases (such as may occur in professional athletes) may require surgery.

13 **A person with a suspected fracture may look pale and clammy and feel faint, dizzy or sick.**
This is usually due to pain but may also be due to internal bleeding caused by the fractured bone, particularly large bones such as the femur or pelvis. Other symptoms of a fracture include swelling or bruising around the site, the limb may be positioned at an unusual angle, the patient may not be able to weight-bear on the limb, or may feel a grinding sensation around the bone. With an open fracture, bleeding will be evident. Irrespective of the type of fracture and where possible, the patient should not be moved until the limb has been immobilized with a splint to prevent movement above and below the fracture site.

14 **Osteoporosis is a metabolic disease of the skeleton characterized by a reduction in bone density.** ✔
Bone is a living tissue that is constantly growing and replacing itself. As the body ages, a certain amount of bone is lost, causing them to become thinner. Thin bones become fragile and more likely to fracture, particularly the bones of the spine, wrist and hips. Osteoporosis happens more commonly in old age when the body becomes less able to replace worn-out bone. It develops slowly with symptoms appearing gradually; early symptoms include pain or difficulty standing/sitting straight (giving the stooping characteristic).

15 **Osteoarthritis can be cured with nonsteroidal anti-inflammatory drugs.** ✗
Osteoarthritis is a chronic and incurable condition, but symptoms can be managed with painkillers, physiotherapy and surgery where necessary. Patients may also be advised to lose weight where appropriate. There can also be variation between extent of joint damage and severity of symptoms. For example, a joint may be severely damaged without causing symptoms, or symptoms may be severe without affecting movement of the joint.

16 **Osteoarthritis is triggered by acute inflammation.**
Osteoarthritis is the most common form of arthritis and is a chronic condition that damages the hyaline (articular) cartilage in joints,

causing secondary damage to the bone, namely development of bony growths and inflammation at the joints. The most affected joints are the knees, hips and small bones in the hands, although any joint may be affected. The degree of disability depends on the site and severity of the cartilage deterioration.

MULTIPLE CHOICE

Correct answers identified in *bold italics*

17 **What type of fracture describes a bone that does not break completely?**

a) stress fracture
b) compression fracture
c) fracture dislocation
d) hairline fracture

A hairline fracture can happen after a trip or fall and can be difficult to detect because the bone is only partially fractured. Stress fractures happen when a bone breaks due to repeated stresses and strains. It is a common complaint in athletes who experience stress fractures in the lower leg or foot bones. Fracture dislocation occurs when the fracture of one of the bones of a joint is accompanied by a dislocation of the same joint. (Avulsion fractures occur when supporting muscle or ligament pulls on the bone, causing it to fracture).

18 **Each of the following represents a type of inflammatory arthritis, with the exception of:**

a) rheumatoid arthritis
b) osteoarthritis
c) lupus
d) osteomyelitis

Inflammatory arthritis relates to joint inflammation caused by an overactive immune system. It usually affects several joints throughout the body at the same time but can also involve a single joint. Inflammatory forms of arthritis are much less common than osteoarthritis, which is the most common type of arthritis caused primarily by mechanical wear and tear of joint areas. Rheumatoid arthritis and lupus represent autoimmune inflammatory conditions that result in joint inflammation and pain. Osteomyelitis can result in septic arthritis and severe inflammation as a result of complications arising from pus discharge into the joint capsule from bone cortex.

19 **Which of the following tests is most commonly used to confirm a fracture?**

a) bone density scan   b) MRI scan

c) CT scan   **d) X-ray**

Fractures are most commonly confirmed using X-ray imaging. If the fracture is more complex (such as comminuted), then further investigations may be made using CT or MRI scanning. Bone density scanning is not useful when investigating fractures because it measures the amount of calcium in the bones. It can be useful in identifying people who are at greater risk of fractures due to low bone density, such as post-menopausal women who have osteoporosis.

20 **Which of the following tests is used to diagnose osteoporosis?**

a) bone density scan   b) CT scan

c) X-ray   d) MRI scan

This is the most accurate measurement of bone density and is used to diagnose osteoporosis. A bone density (dual energy X-ray absorptiometry, DEXA) scan measures the density of bones and compares it to a normal range based on the patient's age and gender. The difference between the patient's bone density and the average is calculated and given a 'T score'. A 'T score' between 0 and 1 = normal; −1 and −2.5 = osteopenia – this indicates the bone density between normal and osteoporosis; osteoporosis is only diagnosed if the 'T score' is below −2.5.

21 **Which of the following is often the first specific symptom of osteoporosis?**

a) unexplained fracture   b) joint pain

c) limb stiffness   d) nerve pain

A sudden, unexplained fracture may be caused by a simple bump or slight fall that would not cause injury in the absence of osteoporosis. Even a cough or a sneeze may cause a rib fracture. Fractured bones in older people can be serious because the bone is no longer able to repair itself effectively, meaning the patient may have a lasting disability that hinders their independence.

22 **Osteoporosis usually affects who?**

a) pregnant women   b) older males

c) children   **d) post-menopausal females**

Osteoporosis is related to the decrease in the hormone oestrogen following the menopause. Oestrogen and testosterone are important hormones for processing calcium, which is essential for bone formation. Males continue to produce testosterone into old age, meaning osteoporosis is less of a risk for older males. Diseases arising in hormone-producing glands, such as diabetes or hypothyroidism, can leave patients at greater risk of osteoporosis.

23 **Which of the following does *not* contribute to carpal tunnel syndrome?**

c) heart failure
a) rheumatoid arthritis

b) renal failure
d) diabetes mellitus

The tendon that passes through the carpal tunnel may become inflamed or fibrous. This causes oedema and compression of the median nerve that runs from the forearm into the hand. Many other conditions that tend to cause fluid retention may also cause swelling in the carpal tunnel, including pregnancy, menopause, hypothyroidism, tuberculosis and benign tumours, as well as oedema due to a bad sprain, dislocation or fracture of the wrist. Symptoms of carpal tunnel syndrome are usually worse at night and in the morning and include pain, burning and paraesthesia (tingling or numbness). Often patients cannot clench the hand in a fist and their skin may be dry and shiny. Pain may spread into the forearm and up into the shoulder, which can sometimes be relieved by shaking the arm vigorously or hanging the arm down the side.

24 **Which of the following drugs are used in treating carpal tunnel syndrome?**

a) morphine
c) paracetamol

b) nonsteroidal anti-inflammatory
d) aspirin

Nonsteroidal anti-inflammatory drugs reduce inflammation around the median nerve, which relieves symptoms. Initially the hand should be rested for 1–2 weeks by splinting the wrist at a neutral angle. If the symptoms are occupation-related, suitable alterations should be made (where possible) to alleviate symptoms. Steroids (cortisone) may be injected into the carpal tunnel to reduce swelling and inflammation around the nerve. Surgical decompression of the median nerve is the last alternative after conservative treatment fails.

25 **Which of the following is not considered an initial symptom of osteoarthritis?**

a) limited movement in affected joints b) pain
c) joint stiffness after wakening **d) *muscle-wasting***

Pain, limited movement and stiffness in moving are considered the main initial symptoms of osteoarthritis and often develop slowly. Other symptoms may develop as the condition progresses, and these include: weakness and muscle-wasting, nodules developing on the joints, joint tenderness, a grating sensation when moving the joint and warmth around the joint – indicating inflammation.

26 **An inability to relax muscles following contraction is a feature of which type of muscular dystrophy?**

a) Duchenne **b) *myotonic***
c) congenital d) limb-girdle

Muscular dystrophy (MD) is descriptive of a group of diseases that cause progressive weakness and loss of muscle mass. Specific signs and symptoms begin at different ages and in different muscle groups, depending on the type of MD. Myotonic MD is characterized by an inability to relax muscles following contractions. The facial and neck muscles are usually the first to be affected. Individuals with this form typically have long, thin faces, drooping eyelids and swan-like necks. Duchenne type MD is the most common form of the disease and is inherited as an X-linked genetic disorder. As such, it is more common in males, although females that have a defective gene present on one of their X chromosomes may present as carriers for the disorder. Signs and symptoms of this type may include frequent falls, large calf muscles, muscle pain and stiffness, and learning disabilities. These signs and symptoms typically appear in early childhood. Congenital MD affects both genders and may be apparent at birth or before age 2 years. Some forms progress slowly and cause only mild disability, while others progress rapidly and cause severe impairment. The hip and shoulder muscles are usually affected first with limb-girdle MD. Individuals with this type of the disease may have difficulty lifting the front part of the foot and are subject to ambulatory problems. Onset usually begins in early childhood. There is no cure for any of these conditions, although medications and therapy can assist in managing symptoms and slowing disease progression.

FILL IN THE BLANKS

27 The most common form of nerve entrapment conditions is *carpal tunnel syndrome*.

Carpal tunnel syndrome (CTS) is a repetitive strain injury resulting from repetitive hand movements that are often occupation-related. It is caused by repeated compression of the median nerve at the wrist. The median nerve is located within the carpal tunnel along with blood vessels and flexor tendons to the fingers and thumb. It is often associated with prolonged keyboard activities such as word-processing. Flexing the wrist is a diagnostic test for carpal tunnel syndrome. If this test produces pain, numbness or tingling, it is likely due to CTS. This test is commonly used in addition to tapping the wrist lightly to see if it produces a tingling feeling or numbness. Together these tests would indicate the median nerve is being compressed and a diagnosis of CTS would be made.

28 A *hernia* occurs when an internal part of the body, such as an organ, pushes through a weakness in the muscle or surrounding tissue wall.

A hernia develops when an organ protrudes abnormally through an opening in a muscular wall. The most common types of hernias are: inguinal, femoral and diaphragmatic. An inguinal hernia occurs when part of the bowel protrudes through the lower abdomen into the groin. It is common among males and people who lift heavy weights, but may also be caused by the physical strain associated with persistent cough or chronic constipation. Femoral hernias occur when fatty tissue or a part of the bowel protrudes into the groin. It is less common than inguinal hernias and more common in females. Hiatus hernia (a form of diaphragmatic hernia) occurs when part of the stomach pushes up into the mediastinum of the chest by squeezing through the oesophageal opening in the diaphragm. It is relatively common and sometimes asymptomatic, although a frequent symptom is heartburn. If a hernia is untreated, it may cause serious complications such as bowel obstruction (depending on location) or it can disrupt blood supply to the surrounding herniated tissue (strangulated hernia). Hernias will not disappear without treatment and due to the risk of these potential complications, they are usually surgically repaired.

29 *Muscular dystrophy* **describes a group of inherited diseases characterized by progressive degeneration of groups of muscles.**
Duchenne muscular dystrophy is the most common form of the condition. It is usually diagnosed around the age of 3 years and generally affects males. Symptoms start in the leg muscles, but quickly advance to other muscle groups. Muscles become progressively weaker and the patient usually dies before the age of 30, often due to cardiac or respiratory failure, when the disorder affects intercostal muscles and/or the diaphragm. Another type of MD is Becker muscular dystrophy, the symptoms of which are similar to those of Duchenne MD. However, they are milder and do not usually appear until a person is 10 or 11 years old, or older. Becker MD progresses more slowly than Duchenne MD and patients usually live a normal lifespan. MD is caused by mutations in the genes for healthy muscle structure and function, causing muscle weakness and progressive disability. The different types of MD are caused by mutations in different genes. Not all types of MD cause severe disability, but there is currently no cure for these conditions.

30 **Approximately 40–60% of patients with osteoarthritis will have a** *genetic* **link.**
Many patients with hand, hip and knee osteoarthritis report family members who have similar symptoms. No gene has yet been identified for the condition. Other risk factors include obesity and previous joint injury. Obesity puts excessive strain on weight-bearing joints, while inadequate healing time after injury or surgery to the joint may also be a contributing factor. People who are at risk of osteoarthritis are encouraged to undertake low-impact weight-bearing exercise such as walking (but not jogging) to strengthen bones. High-impact exercises, like jogging, could cause weak bones to break.

31 **In addition to bisphosphonate drugs, a** *calcium* **supplement may be prescribed if bone density is low.**
A diet rich in calcium (at least 700 mg/day) is recommended to reduce risk of osteoporosis and bone fracture. Patients who are diagnosed with osteoporosis may be prescribed a number of different types of drugs – hormonal and non-hormonal. Previously, hormone replacement therapy (HRT) was prescribed to increase oestrogen levels and therefore enhance calcium absorption, but the adverse side effects associated with prolonged HRT now make it a less popular treatment. Bisphosphonates are non-hormonal drugs

that maintain bone density and reduce fracture rates. Osteoporosis patients are usually recommended to undertake weight-bearing exercise to help increase bone density.

32 | **To treat fractures, the broken bones must first be _aligned_; this is known as 'reducing' the fracture.**

Aligning the bones brings the broken ends together to allow healing. Once correctly aligned, the ends of the broken bone must be held in position, immobilizing the bone while it heals.

PUZZLE GRID

```
33 d              34 o  s  t  35 e  o  m  a  l  a  c  i  a
   i                          p                              36 m     37 g  38 o  u  t
   s        34 a              i                              a   y       s
   l           r              c        41 p     42 t  e  n  d  o  n  i  t  i  s
43 o  s  t  e  44 o  s  a  r  c  o  m  a           k   g        e                    45 b
   c     h     s              n     g  46 f        y   l        o                       u
   a     r     t              d     e     i        l   o        p                       r
   t     o     e              y     t     b        o   b     48 u  r  i  c  a  c  i  d   s
   i     s     o     47 d     l     s     r        s   i        o                       t
   o     c     p        i     i     d     o        i   n        s                       i
   n     o     e        s     t     i     m        s   u        i           49 k        s
         n     i        u     i     s     y            r     50 o  s  t  e  o  a  r  t  h  r  i  t  i  s
         i     a        s     i     a     l            a              y
         a              e     a     l     g                        51 s  p  r  a  i  n
                        a     s     g                  52 o           h
            53 o  s  t  e  o  54 m  y  e  l  i  t  i  s    a        56 t  r  a  n  s  v  e  r  s  e
         55 r           r     o                 a     s  56 t              i
57 m        i        58 c  a  r  p  a  l  t  u  n  n  e  l  o           59 s  t  r  a  i  n
   y        k           h                          o     p
   e        e           y                          n  60 r  h  e  u  m  a  t  o  i  d
   l        t                          i                  y
   o                                   a              62 g
61 m  y  o  s  i  t  i  s                              r  e  e  n  s  t  i  c  k
   a                                62 g              s
```

12 Genetics and hereditary disorders

INTRODUCTION

Genetics is the study of the inheritance of traits passed from parents to their children. Dominant genes will be expressed in any inheritance pattern, while recessive genes will recede to the background – unless both parents carry the recessive gene. The expression of certain genes may also be influenced by environmental factors, for example, height is influenced by parental genes, but also the individual's health and nutrition.

For simple inheritance patterns, it is useful to draw a Punnett square diagram to help understand and determine inheritance probabilities. This is used to calculate the likelihood of inheritance of particular traits.

Genetic disorders arise from changes (mutations) to genes or chromosomes and can also be affected by environmental influences. Disorders can be characterized as autosomal, sex-linked or multifactorial.

Understanding genetics and inherited genetic disorders is an important aspect of healthcare. Nowadays antenatal screening may be offered to pregnant mothers who have an increased risk of having a baby with a genetic or chromosomal abnormality. However, pre-screening counselling is important for these patients, as screening tests are not 100% accurate – they provide an estimate of the likelihood that a foetus has certain conditions. If prenatal screening indicates that a baby has a higher risk, further diagnostic tests may be offered during pregnancy. Many genetic disorders can be identified during pregnancy using diagnostic tests such as amniocentesis or chorionic villus sampling (CVS). The ability to treat and empathize with patients and families affected by genetic and hereditary disorders is an important aspect of the care and support provided by health professionals.

Useful resources

Nurses! Test Yourself in Anatomy and Physiology (2nd edition)
Chapter 13

Ross and Wilson's Anatomy and Physiology in Health and Illness (14th edition)
Chapter 17

Punnett square calculator
http://www.changbioscience.com/genetics/punnett.html

TRUE OR FALSE?

Are the following statements true or false?

| 1 | In autosomal recessive disorders, if both parents are affected with a disorder, their children will also have the condition.

| 2 | Males are more likely to be affected by sex-linked recessive inherited disorders.

| 3 | More than one form of haemophilia exists.

| 4 | Haemophilia can remain undiagnosed into adulthood.

| 5 | Down's syndrome can be cured with gene therapy.

| 6 | The physical signs of Down's syndrome are always detected at birth.

| 7 | Cystic fibrosis is an autosomal dominant disorder.

| 8 | The primary treatment for cystic fibrosis involves managing symptoms.

| 9 | In Huntington's disease, behavioural symptoms often appear before neurological symptoms.

| 10 | The development of some cancers involves the malfunction of certain genes.

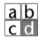 **MULTIPLE CHOICE**

Identify one correct answer for each of the following:

11 If neither parent is affected but both are carriers of a gene for an autosomal recessive disorder, what percentage of children may be affected?
(Hint: it might help to draw a Punnett square).

a) 25%

b) 50%

c) 75%

d) 100%

12 In autosomal recessive disorders, if one parent is affected and the other is a carrier, what percentage of children may be affected?

a) 25%

b) 50%

c) 75%

d) 100%

13 Which of the following is *not* a sex-linked disorder?

a) cystic fibrosis

b) haemophilia

c) Klinefelter's syndrome

d) Turner syndrome

14 In which of the following conditions will affected people have one unpaired X-chromosome?

a) cystic fibrosis

b) haemophilia

c) Klinefelter's syndrome

d) Turner syndrome

15 What type of essential molecule is mutated in cystic fibrosis sufferers, affecting transportation of chloride ions?

a) amino acid

b) carbohydrate

c) lipid

d) vitamin

16 How is Huntington's disease classified?

a) autosomal dominant

b) autosomal recessive

c) multifactorial

d) sex-linked

17 Colour-blindness is classified as:

a) autosomal dominant

b) autosomal recessive

c) dominant, sex-linked

d) recessive, sex-linked

FILL IN THE BLANKS

Fill in the blanks in each statement using the options in this box.
Not all of them are required, so choose carefully!

Turner	diagnostic	dominant
multifactorial	depression	recessive
sex-linked	Fragile X	antidiuretic hormone
chromosomal	desmopressin	screening

18 Down's syndrome is a _____ disorder.

19 Non-invasive prenatal testing is a _____ test available to pregnant woman to estimate risk of certain genetic and chromosomal abnormalities in the foetus.

20 Excessive bleeding experienced by mild haemophilia A patients can be treated by administering the synthetic hormone _____ after injury.

21 Familial hypercholesterolaemia is a _____ inherited disorder.

22 Genetic disorders that are also influenced by environmental/lifestyle factors are called _____ disorders.

23 Loss of personal independence can trigger _____ as a complication of Huntington's disease.

24 Phenylketonuria is an autosomal _____ disorder.

25 _____ ___ syndrome is an inherited learning disability mainly affecting males.

PUZZLE GRID

Use the word bank (below) and clues (overleaf) to solve the puzzle.

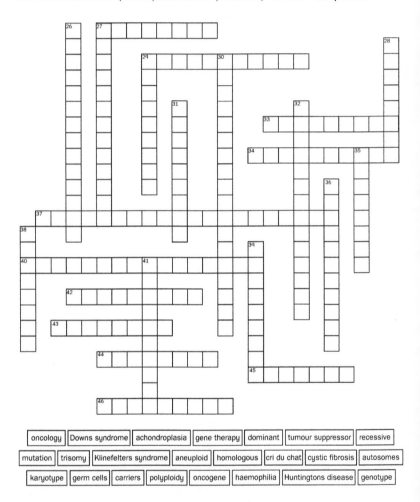

| oncology | Downs syndrome | achondroplasia | gene therapy | dominant | tumour suppressor | recessive |

| mutation | trisomy | Klinefelters syndrome | aneuploid | homologous | cri du chat | cystic fibrosis | autosomes |

| karyotype | germ cells | carriers | polyploidy | oncogene | haemophilia | Huntingtons disease | genotype |

Clues across

27 Expressed version of an allele or gene (8)

29 Experimental technique focusing on the modification or manipulation of DNA expression or to alter the biological properties of living cells for therapeutic use (4, 7)

33 Allele that is manifest only when both copies of a gene have the same genotype (9)

34 Type of chromosomes that pair at meiosis and have the same structural features and pattern of genes (10)

37 Condition that results when a male is born with an extra copy of the X-chromosome; 47 XXY (12, 8)

40 Gene that regulates a cell during cell division and replication (6, 10)

42 Occurrence of one or more extra or missing chromosomes leading to an unbalanced chromosome complement (9)

43 Alleles or variants an individual carries in a particular gene or genetic location; genetic makeup that contributes to the phenotype (8)

44 Mutated form of a gene involved in normal cell growth that in certain circumstances can transform a cell into a tumour cell (8)

45 Chromosomal conditions characterized by possession of an additional chromosome (7)

Clues down

26 Inherited condition that causes sticky mucus to build up in the lungs and digestive system; dysfunction of gene controlling cellular water and chloride transport (6, 8)

27 Genetic disorder caused by the presence of all or part of a third copy of chromosome 21; trisomy 21 (5, 8)

28 Individuals who possess and can pass on a genetic mutation associated with a disease (8)

29 Embryonic cells with the potential of developing into gametes (4, 5)

30 Rare, inherited disease that causes the progressive degeneration of cerebral neurones (11, 7)

31 Any of the numbered chromosomes (as opposed to the sex chromosomes) that control the inheritance of an individual's characteristics except those that are sex-linked (9)

32 Inherited disorder of bone growth that prevents the changing of cartilage (particularly in the long bones of the arms and legs) to bone; form of short-limbed dwarfism (14)

35 Branch of medicine concerned with the diagnosis and treatment of cancer (8)

36 Inherited genetic disorder that impairs the body's ability to make blood clots; factor VIII deficiency (11)

38 Change in a DNA sequence that may result from DNA copying mistakes made during cell division through exposure to radiation, chemicals or infection by viruses (8)

251

Clues across (continued)

46 Diagnostic procedure used to determine chromosomal aberrations in cells; chromosome coding (9)

Clues down (continued)

39 Rare genetic syndrome in which a variable portion of the short arm of chromosome 5 is missing or deleted (3, 2, 4)

41 Lethal chromosome abnormality that may result from polyspermy (10)

ANSWERS

 TRUE OR FALSE?

1 **In autosomal recessive disorders, if both parents are affected with a disorder, their children will also have the condition.**

If both parents are affected, then all their children will definitely be affected with the disorder because there are no unaffected genes in the gene pool. Children can only inherit affected genes from both parents and so will suffer from the disorder.

2 **Males are more likely to be affected by sex-linked recessive inherited disorders.**

Some genetic disorders are caused by genes carried on the X-chromosome, and are known as 'sex-linked' ('X-linked') disorders. Males tend to be affected by recessive sex-linked disorders rather than females because males have only one X-chromosome while females have two. For females to be affected with a recessive sex-linked disorder, they need two copies of the affected gene, although this does not normally happen. Females with one recessive gene will not be affected but will be carriers. Examples of sex-linked disorders include haemophilia, Fragile X syndrome and Klinefelter's syndrome.

3 **More than one form of haemophilia exists.**

There are two forms of the blood clotting disorder, haemophilia: haemophilia A and haemophilia B. The 'classic' form, haemophilia A, affects more that 80% of all sufferers. It is caused by a deficiency or inefficiency of factor VIII, which is essential for blood clotting. The less common form, haemophilia B, is caused by a deficiency or inefficiency in clotting factor IX, which is also involved in the blood clotting cascade.

4 **Haemophilia can remain undiagnosed into adulthood.**

Depending on the severity of the disorder, patients may remain undiagnosed into adulthood. Such patients may not exhibit the characteristic excessive and spontaneous bleeding associated with haemophilia, but may complain of pain or swelling in weight-bearing joints such as the hips, knees and ankles. These patients, classified as mild haemophiliacs, may report prolonged bleeding after surgery or dental extraction, and may exhibit symptoms of internal bleeding or haematuria (blood in urine). Moderate and severe haemophiliacs are usually diagnosed earlier in life. Severe haemophiliacs may exhibit spontaneous bleeding and/or prolonged bleeding after minor trauma. Moderate haemophiliacs can also report excessive bleeding but may not experience regular spontaneous bleeding.

5 | **Down's syndrome can be cured with gene therapy.**
There is no cure for Down's syndrome. However, surgery and hormonal treatments are available to correct or alleviate some of the associated congenital disorders that often accompany the syndrome. Life expectancy is lower than normal and sufferers may have additional learning needs.

6 | **The physical signs of Down's syndrome are always detected at birth.**
The physical signs of Down's syndrome include almond-shaped eyes, protruding tongue, flattened face and small ears. Although the physical characteristics will be present at birth, they are not always detected, especially if the characteristics are not very pronounced. Nevertheless, the diagnosis is usually made shortly after birth. The baby may be born with other abnormalities such as congenital heart disease, cleft lip or palate, clubfoot or duodenal obstruction. Down's syndrome may be diagnosed before birth using chorionic villus sampling (CVS) (between weeks 10 and 13) or amniocentesis (between weeks 15 and 20), although both procedures carry an increased risk of miscarriage. A genetic karyotype (chromosome arrangement analysis) will confirm Down's syndrome by identifying the abnormality on chromosome 21. Alternatively, the quadruple screening test can identify pregnancies that are at greater risk of producing a Down's syndrome (or spina bifida) child, although this test does not provide definitive diagnosis of these conditions.

7 | **Cystic fibrosis is an autosomal dominant disorder.** **X**
Cystic fibrosis (CF) is an autosomal recessive inherited disorder meaning neither parent suffers from CF but if they are *both* carriers of the CF gene, their children have a 25% chance of being affected. In autosomal dominant disorders, at least one parent is affected with the condition and their children will have a 50% chance of

being affected. Examples of autosomal dominant conditions include Huntington's disease and familial hypercholesterolaemia (FH).

8 | **The primary treatment for cystic fibrosis involves managing symptoms.**

As cystic fibrosis (CF) is currently incurable, treatment is focused on maintaining quality of life. Treatments include salt supplements to correct electrolyte imbalance lost through sweat. Patients also take oral pancreatic enzymes to aid digestion since they may be deficient, or the enzymes may be unable to get to the necessary site of action due to the excess mucus in the GI tract. Antibiotics are often prescribed to treat respiratory infections that CF patients are prone to, due to the excess mucus in the respiratory tract. Physiotherapy is often performed on the chest several times a day to remove excess mucus. A mucus-thinning drug (DNase) can be administered, which helps reduce infection and improve lung function. Heart and/ or lung transplant is an option if required (after heart/lung failure). A lot of research is focused on developing gene therapy to replace the faulty gene in CF patients (see Chapter 6, Answer 23).

9 | **In Huntington's disease, behavioural symptoms often appear before neurological symptoms.**

Behavioural symptoms are usually not specific and include hallucination, restlessness, paranoia and mood changes. Since this is an autosomal dominant disorder, people are usually aware of a family history and should seek medical advice as soon as symptoms arise. Neurological symptoms can be similar to those of Parkinson's disease (see Chapter 3, Answers 21, 27).

10 | **The development of some cancers involves the malfunction of certain genes.**

All cancers develop from genetic mutations that cause uncontrolled cell growth. Mutations that affect cell growth can be caused by a number of factors either alone or in combination, namely, environmental factors such as exposure to radiation or certain chemicals. The mutation may occur sporadically or the faulty gene may be inherited but mutates further upon exposure to environmental carcinogens. Inherited mutations in some genes are known to pose an increased risk of certain cancers. Examples include BRCA1/2 mutations, which are strongly associated with an increased risk of breast and/or ovarian cancers, and Lynch syndrome (HNPCC), an autosomal dominant condition that carries a very high risk of colon cancer at a younger age.

MULTIPLE CHOICE

Correct answers identified in *bold italics*

11 **If neither parent is affected but both are carriers of a gene for an autosomal recessive disorder, what percentage of children may be affected?**

a) 25%   b) 50%   c) 75%   d) 100%

Children of two heterozygous parents have a one-in-four chance of being affected (Figure 12.1 – option (4)) with an autosomal recessive disorder such as cystic fibrosis or phenylketonuria (PKU) and a 50% chance of being carriers (Figure 12.1 – options (2), (3)). When one parent is affected but the other is not a carrier (that is, homozygous dominant), no children will be affected with the disorder but will all be carriers (Figure 12.2).

Figure 12.1 Punnett square for cystic fibrosis (both parents are carriers)

♀ Female parent (carrier) \ ♂ Male parent (carrier)	C	c̄
C	(1) CC	(2) Cc̄
c̄	(3) Cc̄	(4) c̄c̄

C = dominant, healthy allele
c̄ = recessive allele associated with CF

Figure 12.2 Punnett square for phenylketonuria inheritance (father not carrier)

Male parent (not carrier) ♀ ♂ Female parent (affected)	P	P
$\bar{p}$	(1) P$\bar{p}$	(2) P$\bar{p}$
$\bar{p}$	(3) P$\bar{p}$	(4) P$\bar{p}$

P = dominant, healthy allele
$\bar{p}$ = recessive allele associated with phenylketonuria

12 | **In autosomal recessive disorders, if one parent is affected and the other is a carrier, what percentage of children may be affected?**

a) 25%　　***b) 50%***　　c) 75%　　d) 100%

Each child will have a one-in-two (50%) chance of being affected with the disorder (Figure 12.3 – options (2), (4)) and a one-in-two (50%) chance of being a carrier of the disorder (Figure 12.3 – options (1), (3)).

Figure 12.3 Punnett square for autosomal recessive inheritance (father carrier)

Male parent (carrier) ♀ ♂ Female parent (affected)	P	p̄
p̄	(1) Pp̄	(2) p̄p̄
p̄	(3) Pp̄	(4) p̄p̄

P = dominant, healthy allele
p̄ = recessive allele associated with disorder

13 **Which of the following is *not* a sex-linked disorder?**

a) *cystic fibrosis*

b) haemophilia

c) Klinefelter's syndrome

d) Turner syndrome

All these conditions are genetic disorders. However, cystic fibrosis is not a sex-linked condition because it is carried on chromosome 7. All the other conditions are inherited through the X-chromosome. Haemophilia is a blood-clotting disorder. Affected people bleed profusely because they are lacking a clotting factor that controls coagulation (see Answers 3, 4). Klinefelter's syndrome is a trisomy condition in males (who have an extra X-chromosome and so have 47 chromosomes), with the sex chromosomes having an XXY arrangement. Turner syndrome is a monosomy sex-linked disorder that affects females. Such patients have only one unpaired X-chromosome, and so they fail to develop and mature as normal females.

14 | **In which of the following conditions will affected people have one unpaired X-chromosome?**

a) cystic fibrosis   b) haemophilia
c) Klinefelter's syndrome   ***d)* Turner syndrome**

Turner syndrome is an unusual sex-linked disorder because it affects females. Affected women are missing an X-chromosome so it is a monosomy condition with only 45 chromosomes in total. Characteristic physical abnormalities include short stature, swelling, broad chest, low hairline, low-set ears and webbed necks. Patients with Turner syndrome typically have non-functioning ovaries, which results in amenorrhoea (absence of menstrual cycle) and sterility. Approximately 98% of foetuses with Turner syndrome are lost through spontaneous miscarriage.

15 | **What type of essential molecule is mutated in cystic fibrosis sufferers, affecting transportation of chloride ions?**

***a)* amino acid**   b) carbohydrate
c) lipid   d) vitamin

Many sufferers of cystic fibrosis have an abnormal ion transport protein resulting from a deletion of three bases that code for the amino acid phenylalanine. The lack of this amino acid affects chloride transport and leads to the formation of thick, sticky mucus in the lungs, digestive tract and other parts of the body. This mucus causes respiratory, metabolic and fertility problems in sufferers and it can often become infected, leaving patients susceptible to frequent respiratory infections (see Chapter 6, Answer 23).

16 | **How is Huntington's disease classified?**

***a)* autosomal dominant**   b) autosomal recessive
c) multifactorial   d) sex-linked

Huntington's disease is an inherited neurodegenerative disease caused by a defect on chromosome 4. It is an autosomal dominant disease because when one parent has Huntington's disease, children will have at least a 50% chance of being sufferers (Figure 12.4). If both parents are affected by the gene, their children have a 75% chance of developing the disease (Figure 12.5 – options (1), (2), (3)). It is extremely rare for the affected parent to be homozygous for the dominant gene (has two affected alleles as in Figure 12.5 – option (1)); in this case, all children will have the dominant gene and therefore will develop the condition.

Figure 12.4 Punnett square for inheritance of Huntington's disease (mother unaffected)

♀ Female parent (unaffected) \ ♂ Male parent (affected)	H	h
h	(1) Hh	(2) hh
h	(3) Hh	(4) hh

H = dominant, disease-causing allele
h = recessive, normal allele

Figure 12.5 Punnett square for inheritance of Huntington's disease (both parents affected)

♀ Female parent (affected) \ ♂ Male parent (affected)	H	h
H	(1) HH	(2) Hh
h	(3) Hh	(4) hh

H = dominant, disease-causing allele
h = recessive, normal allele

17 **Colour-blindness is classified as:**

a) autosomal dominant
b) autosomal recessive
c) dominant, sex-linked
d) recessive, sex-linked

Colour-blindness (colour vision deficiency) is a recessive trait that affects the function of cells in the retina of the eye that detect colours and therefore reduces the ability of the affected individual to interpret colours. Most of the genes involved in colour vision are transmitted on the X-chromosome, thus it is a recessive, sex-linked condition that mainly affects males. A colour-blind male will pass his recessive gene for the condition to all female children who will carry the recessive gene (Figure 12.6 – options (1), (3)).

Figure 12.6 Punnett square for sex-linked inheritance of colour-blindness (father affected, mother carrier)

Male parent (affected) ♀ ♂ Female parent (carrier)	X$\bar{c}$	Y
XC	(1) XC X$\bar{c}$	(2) XC Y
X$\bar{c}$	(3) X$\bar{c}$ X$\bar{c}$	(4) X$\bar{c}$ Y

XC = dominant allele for normal colour vision carried on X-chromosome
X$\bar{c}$ = recessive allele for colour-blindness, carried on X-chromosome
Y = normal Y (male) chromosome that carries no gene for colour vision

The sons of a female carrier have a 50% chance of being affected. (Figure 12.7 – option (4)).

Figure 12.7 Punnett square for sex-linked inheritance of colour-blindness (mother carrier)

Female parent (carrier) \\ Male parent (unaffected) ♀ ♂	XC	Y
XC	(1) XC XC	(2) XC Y
XC̄	(3) XC XC̄	(4) XC̄ Y

XC = dominant allele for normal colour vision carried on X-chromosome
XC̄ = recessive allele for colour-blindness, carried on X-chromosome
Y = normal Y (male) chromosome that carries no gene for colour vision

The most common form of the disorder (about 95%) is red–green colour-blindness where sufferers cannot distinguish between red and green. Less than 5% of sufferers cannot distinguish between blue and yellow, while the rarest form of the disorder is 'true' colour-blindness when no colours are detected and everything is interpreted as black, white and shades of grey (these patients have poor vision and are very light-sensitive). Diagnosis is usually via a series of tests involving coloured dots and although there is no cure, most sufferers adapt very well and lead normal lives (red–green colour blind people are permitted to drive in most countries).

FILL IN THE BLANKS

18 **Down's syndrome is a _chromosomal_ disorder.**
Also called Trisomy 21, Down's syndrome is caused by an extra chromosome 21, which means people with the condition have a total of 47 chromosomes (instead of 46). It is strongly associated

with the age of the mother, being more common in children born to mothers over 35 years. This is thought to be caused by changes to the ova as the woman ages.

19 **Non-invasive prenatal testing is a _screening_ test available to pregnant women to estimate risk of certain genetic and chromosomal abnormalities in the foetus.**

Non-invasive prenatal testing (NIPT) (also known as non-invasive prenatal screening, or NIPS) is available to pregnant women who wish to determine the risk that their baby will be born with certain genetic or chromosomal abnormalities, such as Down's syndrome (Trisomy 21), Edwards' syndrome (Trisomy 18) and Patau's syndrome (Trisomy 13). This test analyses small fragments of DNA circulating in the mother's bloodstream by taking a sample of blood from the woman's arm. Unlike most DNA, which is found inside the nucleus of a cell, these fragments – called cell-free DNA (cf-DNA) – are free-floating and not found inside cells. For this reason, NIPT screening is considered relatively safe for both mother and baby, and it is also considered to be very accurate, although it must be remembered that no screening test is 100% accurate.

20 **Excessive bleeding experienced by mild haemophilia A patients can be treated by administering the synthetic hormone _desmopressin_ after injury.**

Desmopressin is usually administered intravenously and works by stimulating the production of clotting factor VIII. It can produce side effects, including headache and nausea. Desmopressin is not as effective at treating mild haemophilia B because this form is caused by a lack of clotting factor IX. Haemophilia B can be treated with the drug nonacog alfan. Moderate and severe haemophiliacs will be treated prophylactically.

21 **Familial hypercholesterolaemia is a _dominant_ inherited disorder.**

Familial hypercholesterolaemia (FH) is characterized by high levels of low-density lipoprotein (LDL) cholesterol in the blood, which leaves patients at greater risk of developing cardiovascular diseases at a younger age. Since it is a dominant inherited disorder, it is quite common, occurring in around one-in-500 people. Children of those affected have a 50% chance of being affected themselves. Affected individuals will have elevated serum cholesterol readings and should have their levels monitored regularly. These patients are usually prescribed statins to help reduce the levels of LDL in the blood by reducing the amount of cholesterol naturally produced by the liver. Patients are also encouraged to make lifestyle adjustments to reduce their risk of developing cardiovascular diseases.

22 **Genetic disorders that are also influenced by environmental/ lifestyle factors are called *multifactorial* disorders.**

One example of a multifactorial disorder is a cleft lip or a cleft palate. Multifactorial genetic disorders can be very complex. Along with genetic factors, there are lifestyle factors that can contribute to these conditions such as maternal smoking and alcohol consumption, as well as maternal obesity and lack of folic acid in the diet during early pregnancy. Cleft conditions are usually treated successfully with surgery and sometimes require speech therapy. Neural tube defects (spina bifida) are also considered multifactorial disorders and are associated with diets low in folic acid.

23 **Loss of personal independence can trigger *depression* as a complication of Huntington's disease.**

As the disease progresses, patients will need assistance and supervision, eventually requiring 24-hour care. This loss of independence can lead to depression. Patients often report having witnessed the devastating effects on a family member who previously suffered with the disease. Knowledge of how devastating the disease is can be a major cause of depression and even suicide. Depression is a common problem among sufferers of genetic and inherited disorders, particularly patients who lack personal independence.

24 **Phenylketonuria is an autosomal *recessive* disorder.**

Phenylketonuria (PKU) is an inherited recessive disorder (see Figures 12.2 and 12.3) that develops when the body cannot synthesize the enzyme required to convert the amino-acid phenylalanine to tyrosine. This conversion is necessary to prevent an accumulation of phenylalanine in the body, since it is toxic in large amounts, causing irreversible damage to many organs. There is no cure for PKU, although all newborns in the UK are screened for the disorder (during the heel-prick test), usually at 5 days old. Treatment is mainly dietary where sufferers who adhere to a strict diet (limiting phenylalanine intake) can lead relatively normal lives.

25 | ***Fragile X* syndrome is an inherited learning disability mainly affecting males.**

Fragile X syndrome is a dominant sex-linked disorder that causes a spectrum of characteristic physical, intellectual, emotional and behavioural features that range from severe to mild. It accounts for the majority of learning disabilities affecting males. Physical symptoms include long face, large ears and flat feet. A range of emotional and behavioural symptoms will be present, including shyness, an inability to make eye contact and obsessive behaviours. Some individuals with Fragile X syndrome also meet the diagnostic criteria for autistic spectrum disorders (ASDs). Although rare in females, those who have the syndrome experience symptoms to a lesser degree because of their second X-chromosome. Fragile X syndrome can be diagnosed during pregnancy by amniocentesis. There is no cure for the condition and affected individuals are recommended for educational and behavioural therapies.

PUZZLE GRID

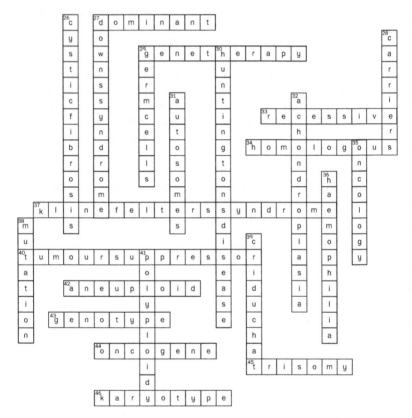

Glossary

Aetiology: the study of causes of disease.

Apoptosis: a normal part of cell development when the cell undergoes programmed cell death through a series of biochemical changes in the cell. The cell debris from apoptosis does not cause harm to the adjacent cells; this is how it differs from necrosis.

Bradycardia: slow heartbeat, usually less than 60 beats per minute in a resting adult.

Bradykinesia: slowness of movement.

Cardiac arrhythmia: abnormal electrical activity in the heart. The heart beat may be too fast or too slow and may be regular or irregular.

Cyanosis: blue/purple discoloration of the skin and mucous membranes, characteristic of hypoxia.

Dysaesthesia: numbness or tingling ('pins and needles').

Dysphagia: difficulty swallowing.

Dyspnoea: shortness of breath, breathlessness.

Dysuria: painful urination.

Fatigue: tiredness, weariness.

Glycosuria: (or glucosuria) glucose in the urine.

Gram's stain: a staining technique used to classify bacteria. Gram-positive bacteria retain the violet stain; Gram-negative bacteria do not.

Haematuria: blood in urine, usually arising from the kidneys.

Haemodilution: increase in plasma volume in the blood, which consequently dilutes the concentration of red blood cells.

Hypercalcaemia: elevated calcium levels in the blood.

Hypercapnia: increased concentration of carbon dioxide in the blood.

Hyperglycaemia: excessively high blood glucose levels (indicates uncontrolled diabetes).

Hyperkalaemia: high potassium levels in the blood.

Hypermagnesaemia: high levels of magnesium in the blood – can occur in renal failure when patients are given excess laxatives or antacids; can also be caused by enemas.

Hyperphosphataemia: elevated levels of phosphate in the blood – common in chronic kidney disease.

Hypersecretion: excess secretion.

Hypertension: high blood pressure – usually describes *persistent* high blood pressure.

Hyperthermia: excessively high core body temperature, usually caused by sunstroke or overwhelming bacterial infection.

Hyperthyroidism: overactive thyroid, secreting excess thyroid hormones.

Hyperventilate: over-breathing; when breathing is faster and deeper than necessary (causing excessive carbon dioxide to be exhaled).

Hypervolaemia: (or fluid overload) abnormally increased volume of blood, most commonly due to congestive heart failure.

Hypocalcaemia: low serum calcium levels, possibly due to vitamin D deficiency.

Hypocapnia: abnormally low levels of carbon dioxide in the blood.

Hypoglycaemia: low blood glucose (sugar) levels, possibly due to the administration or secretion of too much insulin.

Hypokalaemia: low potassium levels in the blood, which can be caused by diuretics and laxatives.

Hypomagnesaemia: low levels of magnesium in the blood – often refers to systemic magnesium deficiency, can be caused by chronic diarrhoea or alcoholism.

Hypoperfusion: decreased blood flow through an organ or tissue.

Hypophosphataemia: abnormally low levels of phosphate in the blood – common in malnutrition.

Hyposecretion: decrease in secretion or release of a substance.

Hypotension: abnormally low blood pressure.

Hypothermia: excessively low core body temperature.

Hypothyroidism: under-active thyroid, secreting insufficient thyroxine.

Hypovolaemia: decreased volume of circulating blood (specifically blood plasma), which may be due to dehydration, haemorrhage, excessive diarrhoea or diuretic drugs.

Hypoxia: lack of oxygen.

Ischaemia: decreased blood supply to organ or tissue.

Lethargy: tiredness, sluggishness.

Metastasis: movement of malignant cells from one location in the body to another, usually via the blood or lymphatic system.

Necrosis: an undesirable form of cell death usually caused by factors external to the cell, such as trauma, toxins or infection. Gangrene is an example of a dangerous accumulation of necrotic tissue.

Nocturia: frequent urination at night.

Pallor: pale in colour.

Palpate: examination of the body by touching or pressing with the fingers or the palm of the hand.

Palpitation: excessive beating of the heart.

Pathogen: disease-causing agent or microorganism.

Pathophysiology: changes to the normal anatomy and physiology due to illness or disease.

Polydipsia: excessive thirst.

Polyphagia: increased appetite.

Polyuria: excessive urination.

Post-prandial: after eating.

Pre-prandial: before eating.

Proteinuria: protein in the urine.

Reperfusion: restoration of blood flow to an organ or tissue – for example, after MI or CVA.

Resistance: opposition to airflow in the lungs or chest wall.

Septicaemia: blood poisoning, sepsis, septic shock.

Tachycardia: rapid heartbeat, usually more than 100 beats per minute in a resting adult.

Urticaria: hives.

Vasoconstriction: narrowing of blood vessels due to contraction of smooth muscle surrounding the walls; reduces blood flow (commonly caused by increased calcium concentration in cells).

Vasodilation: widening of blood vessels due to relaxation of smooth muscle surrounding the walls; increases blood flow (decrease in blood pressure).